Praise

'A book to help us choose hope.'

Iona Heath, British Medical Journal

'After reading this book, I do believe that literature can engender a sense of deep empathy and compassion.'

Austin O'Carroll, British Journal of General Practice

'I was particularly moved by Frances's reaction to the Gerard Manley Hopkins poems, by the author's discernment that those poems were probably right for that patient at that time and his courage in trusting his professional and personal instincts in employing them as part of her treatment.'

Alan Brough, actor, television and radio host, and comedian based in Australia

Reading to Stay Alive

Reading to Stay Alive: Tolstoy, Hopkins and the Dilemma of Existence

Christopher Dowrick

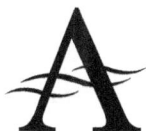

ANTHEM PRESS

Anthem Press
An imprint of Wimbledon Publishing Company
www.anthempress.com

This edition first published in UK and USA 2024
by ANTHEM PRESS
75–76 Blackfriars Road, London SE1 8HA, UK
or PO Box 9779, London SW19 7ZG, UK
and
244 Madison Ave #116, New York, NY 10016, USA

First published in the UK and USA by Anthem Press in 2022

British Library Cataloguing-in-Publication Data
A catalogue record for this book is available from the British Library.

Library of Congress Cataloging-in-Publication Data
A catalog record for this book has been requested.

ISBN-13: 978-1-83999-181-3 (Pbk)
ISBN-10: 1-83999-181-X (Pbk)

This title is also available as an e-book.

Books are possibilities. They are escape routes. They give you options when you have none. Each one can be a home for an uprooted mind.

Matt Haig, *Reasons to Stay Alive* (London: Canongate, 2015), 242

In memory of Amanda Mitchell-Haynes

CONTENTS

Figures   xi

Acknowledgements   xii

1. Staying Alive?   1
    Five Stories   1
    Suicidal Ideas and Actions   4
    Caring for People with Suicidal Thoughts   6
    Acknowledge the Deeply Unconsolable   8
    Themes of This Book   14
    Perspectives   15
    Notes   16

2. Thwarted Belongingness   19
    Anomie and Alienation   19
    Melancholia and Thanatos   21
    Social Roots of Suicide   23
    Belonging and Burden   25
    Defeat and Entrapment   27
    Sense of Safety   30
    Suicide as a Communicative Act   32
    Informing Literary Reading   32
    Notes   33

3. Escape from Them All and from Myself   37
    It's All So Unimportant   38
    So as Not to Be Ashamed   40
    You Will Regret This   45
    The Zest Is Gone   47
    He Acted and Lived Unfalteringly and Definitely   51
    Serving the Universe   54
    Notes   57

4. Not Choose Not to Be   61
    Simple and Beautiful Oneness   62
    A Continually Jaded and Harassed Mind   64
    My Lament Is Cries Countless   66
    It Brings a Closeness   70
    Can Something, Hope   73
    Leave Comfort Root-Room   76
    Plough Down Sillion Shine   79
    Notes   81

5. Points of Transformation   85
    An Everyday Temptation   86
    A Denial of Experience   88
    Prate Not to Me of Suicide   91
    The Artist Must Play   93
    I Can't Wrap This Up   96
    What Good Is Done?   99
    And Then We Shall Dwell Together   102
    Points of Transformation   106
    Notes   107

6. Creating *Raisons d'etre*   111
    A Vain, Fruitless, and Self-Contradictory Effort   112
    Intentional Entity   116
    Desire Is the Very Essence of Man   118
    Vastly More Intersubjectivity   122
    The Struggle Towards the Heights   124
    Continually Completely New?   126
    Notes   128

7. Staying Alive   131
    Sunt Lacrimae Rerum   132
    Back to Black   136
    Final Reflections   138
    Notes   139

Index   141

FIGURES

1.1   The P4 screener   7
2.1   Interpersonal theory of suicide model   25
2.2   Integrated motivational-volitional model of suicidal behaviour   28
2.3   Sense of safety: whole person domains   31

ACKNOWLEDGEMENTS

Phil Davis inspired me to write this book. Megan Greiving, Jebaslin Hephzibah and Sreejith Govindan ensured its completion.

Amongst the many people – family and friends, patients, academics, clinicians – who have kindly offered me their advice, comment, criticism and guidance, or allowed me to refer to their personal narratives, I specifically wish to thank Andrew Bennett, Josie Billington, Colette Brannan, Simon Capewell, Amy Chandler, Anna and Clare Dowrick, Stefan Hjørleifsson, Leigh Holmes, Mandy Johnstone, Bryony, Richard and Star Kendall, Daniel Lawrence, Anne MacFarlane, Susan Martin, Carl May, David Misselbrook, Faraz Mughal, Rory O'Connor, Mary and Tomas O'Reilly-deBrún, Teresa Pearson, Stephen Poole, Joanne Reeve, Peter Riley, Emmert Roberts, Malcolm and Rachel Savage, William Wootten and Emily Yue.

I am grateful to Dougal Jeffries for his constructive review of the full manuscript.

Permissions

Chapter 1

STAYING ALIVE?

Five Stories

Charlie used to be the singer in a band. She felt beautiful then. I'm told she had a wonderful voice, alternative folk and rhythm and blues, and could render a fine version of Joan Armatrading's *Love and Affection*.

But that was a long time ago, before she met Ken. Before endless years of controlling, contempt and manipulation. Before constant criticism and belittling, frequently aimed at her Black heritage. Before she provided him with three children, kept an immaculate household, cooked and washed and tidied. But it was never enough, she was never good enough. He refused to marry her; she was not worth the effort or the expense.

Then came breast cancer, and a double mastectomy. Ken declined to visit her in hospital, lost any residual interest in their sex life and blatantly started an affair in work.

Charlie tried to leave him, several times, but kept on being drawn back, feeling unworthy to live on her own. Alcohol, usually vodka, dulled the pain.

Finally, with encouragement from her many good friends, she moved out and rented her own place. Her sense of self began, slowly, to flourish. She rediscovered her passion for Liverpool Football Club, and her fascination with the parallel universes in Michael Moorcock's science fiction novels. Life was better, especially now her granddaughter Tammy was on the scene. Charlie had a purpose again, a reason for living.

But not for long.

The cancer comes roaring back, now with secondaries in her spine and liver. Vodka helps dull this pain too, but only for a while. Her vulnerabilities resurface, and she takes an overdose of venlafaxine and co-codamol. Her son is furious with her, and stops all contact with Tammy.

Then the COVID-19 pandemic strikes. Charlie is living alone and at high risk of infection, so has to self-isolate completely for weeks on end.

The fear and loneliness become too much for her. She takes another overdose, and keeps on drinking. She reaches out to her son in the hope of a few seconds conversation with Tammy, but her call is blocked.

Frances looks immaculate. She is polite and understated. She is always on time for her appointments with me and never seeks to extend them beyond the allotted 10 or 15 minutes. She has worked with the civil service for many years and now holds a senior position in the Home Office. She lives alone with her cat, Danny. She attends her local Catholic church regularly, and finds comfort in her faith. She has a few friends, mostly through work; she is good at helping them with their problems but doesn't talk much about herself.

Yet Frances finds life immensely difficult. She describes it as a never-ending, bleak monotony. Each day she has to make an enormous effort of will, first to get up and then to keep going. Like Eleanor Rigby, wearing the face that she keeps in a jar by the door. If it were not for Danny, her faith and her work (in that order), she is not sure it would be worth the effort of staying alive.

I do not know much about her early life, as she is guarded about the information she discloses. She was born in Ireland, the only child of older parents. She tells me her father was devoted to her but died when Frances was 9 or 10; after that, her mother was too wrapped up in her own grief to take much notice of her. I wonder about other adverse events in her formative years. I know she has been under the care of mental health teams in the past, had psychotherapy for a while and spent at least one period as an in-patient on a psychiatric ward.

We agree to meet every few weeks. I think she finds it helpful to share – however tentatively – some of her despair with me. Maybe she feels a little less alone after our conversations. She has no interest in being referred for further counselling. We discuss antidepressant medication, but she has a cardiac arrhythmia which renders that problematic. She starts a gratitude diary, each evening writing down three things that she has appreciated during the day. She brings this in to show me every time we meet: Danny features strongly. We discover a common interest in literary reading: she lends me a novel about the Sufi mystic Rumi, and I introduce her to the poetry of Gerard Manley Hopkins.

We are making some gentle progress, when two problems arise. Following a major civil service restructure, Frances is made redundant from work at very short notice. And Danny develops severe, possibly life-threatening kidney problems.

I first met Darren when he was 19, with piercings through lip, nose and eyebrows, and scarring up both arms. He told me about parental separation, fostering and emotional abuse, bullying in school; how cutting himself with a razor relieved his psychic pain, at least for a few minutes; how booze kept him from feeling too much but often led to fights with friends, nightclub doormen and police. His only comfort was beating the hell out of his drum kit in the middle of the night. He didn't think he'd live much longer, and I feared he might be right.

Behind his angry ranting I heard a lost, lonely and frightened little boy. I wanted to give him a huge hug and bring him home with me, but I contented myself with a friendly smile, a warm handshake and an agreement to meet again soon. I committed myself to seeing him regularly, and offered him the options of psychotropic medication and a referral to our local community mental health team.

Darren came to see me every few weeks over the next few years. He stayed alive. He still mostly ranted, and I still mostly listened, but there was less booze and fewer fights in his life. He started a relationship with Mark, who lives with him on and off. He rescued an Alsatian dog, Koda, to whom he becomes utterly devoted. His drumming skills found outlet in two local bands – one with a possible recording contract. Beneath the anguish, I discover a young man with a keen critical intelligence, great compassion for his family and friends, and an utter disdain for what he sees as so much rhetorical 'political bullshit'. He is determined to live his life genuinely, whatever the cost.

But recently, Darren's life has become more difficult again. He disagrees with the musical direction of the band with the recording contract and they have parted company. He has money worries and is involved with endless arguments with the benefits agency. His partner is still around, but Mark has a lot of problems of his own and they are finding it difficult to get along together.

Then Koda dies....

All three of these people, Charlie, Frances and Darren, are now at critical points in their lives. They are each in a dilemma. They are in a state of uncertainty, faced with two equally unfavourable options, a situation in which a difficult choice has to be made. The question of whether or not to stay alive is real, practical and immediate. There is no clear or compelling reason why any of them should do so.

The same was true, a while ago, for both Leo and Gerard.

Leo was born to a wealthy Russian landowning family, apparently with a silver spoon in his mouth. But his mother died when he was only two, after giving birth to his younger sister, and he missed her horribly. His father died (possibly of a stroke, possibly by poison) seven years later. He was looked after by a series of relatives, some of whom cared for him more than others, and moved house several times during his childhood. From adolescence, he considered himself to be physically unattractive and he found it difficult to make lasting relationships. He greatly admired his older brother Nicholas and was devastated when he died of tuberculosis. Leo spent time in the army, gambling excessively, before embarking on a life as an educator and writer.

Eventually, Leo marries and settles in a comfortable property in the countryside, garnering major literary success and 14 children along the way. But he is frequently overwhelmed by a sense of futility, and frustrated by the pointlessness of his existence:

> Had I simply understood that life has no meaning I might have accepted it peacefully, knowing that that was my lot. But I could not be calmed by this. Had I been like a man in a wood from which he knows there is no way out, I might have been able to live; but I was like a man in a wood who is lost, and terrified by this rushes around hoping to find his way out, knowing with each step he is getting more lost, and yet unable to stop rushing about.
>
> It was all quite dreadful. And so, in order to escape from this horror, I wanted to kill myself.[1]

Leo becomes so worried about his inability to resist his desire to die by suicide that he gives up his favourite pastime of duck shooting, for fear that he will turn his gun on himself.

Brought up in a conventional middle-class family in London, Gerard becomes a poet and a priest. After spending time as a parish priest in Liverpool (just a stone's throw from my University office), he is sent by his religious order to Dublin, with the task of teaching Latin and Greek to students who he feels show little interest or aptitude for these subjects, preparing and grading apparently endless examination papers. He feels alienated, from his students, from his home and from his friends. He worries about the threat of revolution in Ireland, following recent demonstrations and political assassinations, and fears for his personal safety.

Gerard experiences the most intense loneliness: 'To seem the stranger lies my lot, my life/ Among strangers'. He writes to his good friend Robert of 'work, worry and a languishment of body and mind', with 'fits of sadness' that 'resemble madness'.[2] In the midst of despair, his poetry – previously full of joy in the natural world and compassion for his fellow men – becomes terrible and dark. 'What hours, O what black hoùrs we have spent/ This night!' 'O the mind, mind has mountains; cliffs of fall/ Frightful, sheer, no-man-fathomed'. He wrestles with his God, and with persisting thoughts of suicide.

Suicidal Ideas and Actions

These stories are all true: the first three are based on a number of patients I have known, with their names and biographical details altered for reasons of confidentiality. Sadly, they are far from unusual or unique.

Suicide may be formally defined as 'an act with fatal outcome, which the deceased, knowing or expecting a fatal outcome, has initiated and carried out with the purpose of bringing about wanted changes'.[3] The word 'wanted' here indicates the presence of a degree of intention with regard to the act. Understood on this basis, it is the cause of about 1.5 per cent of all deaths:[4] that equates to about 800,000 people every year, of which almost 80 per cent are from low- and middle-income countries.[5] And each suicide affects a large circle of people who knew the person concerned, and may be in need of clinical services or support following exposure.[6]

But this is only the tip of the iceberg, a tiny proportion of all the people who have ever wondered whether or not it is worth staying alive. Thoughts, plans and acts of suicide or self-harm are common. In an English survey conducted in 2014 with over 7,500 people aged 16 or above, more than one in five (20.6 per cent) reported they had thought of taking their own life at some point; this was more common in women than men, and in people of working age than those aged 65 or more.[7] A study across 17 countries, involving interviews with almost 85,000 people, found that almost 1 in 10 (9.2 per cent) had considered suicide at some time in their lives; 3.1 per cent had made plans to kill themselves and 2.7 per cent had actually attempted to do so. In this international survey, the main risk factors for suicidal ideas were being female, younger, less educated or unmarried; and having a mental disorder.[8]

Taking people's ideas of suicide or self-harm in any given year, we find that during 2015 almost ten million adults in the United States thought seriously about trying to kill themselves, including 2.7 million who made suicide plans and 1.4 million who made a nonfatal suicide attempt. These numbers mean that 4.0 per cent of adults in the United States had serious thoughts of suicide, 1.1 per cent made suicide plans and 0.6 per cent attempted suicide during that year.[9]

More generally, it is very common for us to have, at times, a preference for not staying alive. In the United Kingdom, during the first lockdown in response to the COVID-19 pandemic in the spring of 2020, more than 85,000 people (including me) responded to a weekly national survey. Consistently between March and May, more than 10 per cent of us reported 'thoughts that you would be better off dead or of hurting yourself in some way'.

Thoughts of death or self-harm were at least twice as common amongst younger people, those living alone, those with a lower household income, and at least three times as common amongst people with a diagnosed mental health condition.[10] For me, in none of those categories, my main thoughts – occasional, not persistent – were that life was just so difficult that it might be easier not to be around anymore. They were prompted by at times almost overwhelming worry about the effects of COVID on me and my loved ones; and relieved by a combination of support from family and close friends, endorphin-generating half-marathon training runs, Charlie Mackesy's cartoons, and absorption in Hilary Mantel's *The Mirror and the Light*.

Caring for People with Suicidal Thoughts

One of my most crucial tasks as a family doctor is to assess my patients' risk of suicide, especially if they are experiencing mental health problems such as depression. It is so important to explore this – sensitively – with patients.

This whole topic can be troubling and distressing. I still vividly remember, more than 20 years later, two of my patients who killed themselves: one was certainly in part my fault, when I gave a young man a full month's prescription for a tricyclic antidepressant without making any attempt to assess his suicide risk; the other was a complete and devastating surprise, a talented young photographer whom I believed I had successfully helped to negotiate her way out of a difficult relationship.

Many health and social care professionals feel unprepared to manage suicide, and hence tend to shy away from it.[11] Current trends in professional divisions of labour, and the increasingly transactional nature of general practice consultations, make it too easy for us to ignore profound distress and appear indifferent to the suffering of our patients.[12] Some of us may also be disconcerted by our own ideas and impulses towards self-harm, and perhaps have a subconscious motivation to keep the subject taboo.

Even when we acknowledge the problem of suicide, we may find it challenging to make sense of a problem which is not clearly biomedical in nature, or to grapple with ideas of social and psychological causes.[13] We may worry that discussing self-harm will increase the risk of patients acting on these impulses. There is no evidence that this is the case.[14] Only by understanding what our patients' risk is, can we hope to offer them the right support, help and treatment to meet their needs.

We can consider suicide risk in four related dimensions. First is *intent*, whether the patient has thoughts of ending their life or harming themselves. Are these thoughts general, in the sense of wishing to no longer be alive, or are they more specific, in terms of a definite desire to die? Second are *plans*, whether they have specific ideas about how they will kill themselves and, related to that, whether they have access to the means to carry these plans out. So, for example, a plan to end their life by shooting themselves will depend, as Leo realised, on having access to a gun, while a plan to take a lethal overdose of sleeping pills or pain killers, perhaps in combination with alcohol, will depend on having access to prescription medication. Third are *actions*, both past and current. Has the patient tried to kill themselves previously, either in the distant past or more recently? And fourth is *prevention*. What, if anything, is stopping them from acting on their suicidal thoughts? Protective factors will vary from person to person, but common ones include a strong religious faith, family support to find alternative solutions to their problems, having children at home, a sense of responsibility for others and problem-solving skills.[15]

Alternatively, we may approach suicide risk by assessing the '4 Ps' – *past* suicide attempts, suicide *plan*, *probability* of completing suicide and *preventive* factors. There is a simple screening measure that we can use to help us make this assessment, which provides a classification of minimal, lower and higher risk based upon responses to these four items (Figure 1.1).[16]

There are many well-established therapeutic strategies available to family doctors and other front-line care professionals, which have the underlying purpose of increasing a sense of hope, reducing the power of suicidal thoughts and maximising the power of the individual not to act on them. These include developing a safety plan,[17] managing and treating any underlying illness, removing access to lethal means (e.g., by prescribing medication in small amounts) and working collaboratively not only with patients but also with

Have you had thoughts of actually hurting yourself?

NO   YES

| 4 Screening Questions |

1. Have you ever attempted to harm yourself in the past?

NO   YES

2. Have you thought about how you might actually hurt yourself?

NO   YES → [How? _____]

3. There's a big difference between having a thought and acting on a thought. How likely do you think it is that you will act on these thoughts about hurting yourself or ending your life some time over the next month?

a. Not at all likely _____
b. Somewhat likely _____
c. Very likely _____

4. Is there anything that would prevent or keep you from harming yourself?

NO   YES → [What? _____]

| Risk Category | Shaded ("Risk") Response | |
	Items 1 and 2	Items 3 and 4
Minimal	Neither is shaded	Neither is shaded
Lower	At least 1 item is shaded	Neither is shaded
Higher		At least 1 item is shaded

Figure 1.1 The P4 screener.

carers and other health and social care professionals. We also have potentially valuable roles to play in supporting people bereaved by suicide.[18]

If you are a care professional and wish to know more about these important approaches, there are two helpful primary care textbooks: the second edition of Linda Gask's *Primary Care Mental Health*;[19] and Gabriel Ivbijaro's *Companion to Primary Care Mental Health*.[20] The World Health Organisation also has valuable information for primary care practitioners in its *mhGAP intervention Guide*,[21] and for policy makers in *Live Life*, its guide for suicide prevention.[22] And for people struggling with their own thoughts of suicide, or trying to help someone who is vulnerable, I recommend Matt Haig's *Reasons to Stay Alive*,[23] and *When It Is Darkest* by Rory O'Connor.[24]

However, my intention with this book is to investigate a different set of perspectives, combining my longstanding commitment to good mental health with my belief in the healing power of literature. I have previously explored ways in which literary reading can inform our understanding and our approach to those perceptions and emotions commonly related to current concepts of the depressive experience.[25,26] Here I have a more specific purpose, to consider how literary reading may ameliorate our personal and vicarious experiences of suicidal ideas and actions. I hope that my investigation will be of value not only to scholars interested in the intersections between literature and health, but also directly – and more importantly – to people facing their own dilemmas of existence, as well as their families and friends, and the care professionals with whom they make purposeful contact.

Acknowledge the Deeply Unconsolable

There is recurring controversy about the healing or destructive power of literature. As those of you with an historical interest may already know, way back in classical Greece, in the fourth-century BCE, a major argument erupted about the safety or otherwise of imitating tragic events, in which human actions have severe, often dire consequences, in theatre and poetry. As Friedrich Nietzsche tellingly commented, this debate boiled down to the enduring conflict between our reason and our desires, symbolised on the one hand by Apollo, god of truth and rationality, and on the other by Dionysus, god of wine and wild emotions.[27] Homer's *Iliad* with its heroic and tragic tales of the Trojan wars was the main case in point.

Plato was worried that dramatic poetry, especially tragedy, inflamed the passions and was a danger to civic order. He believed that the imaginary depiction of events leading to sorrow and happiness causes needless distress and excitement in the audience. It numbs our faculties of reason, paralyses balanced thought and encourages our baser impulses. It waters and nourishes feelings that ought to be allowed to dry up. A man should bear his apparent misfortunes, such as the loss of a son, with dignity and fortitude; indeed, if he is capable of it he should not grieve at all. Dramatic poetry has no healthy function, and – in stark contrast to the positive attributes of philosophy – cannot be called good. This is not simply a question of psychological health, but more broadly part of the failure of the soul to see the truth about the good. Our reason will tell the soul that life is not worth much in any case, and certainly not worth getting excited about. Plato's conclusion was that the dramatic poet should be banned:

> And so we may now with justice refuse to allow him entrance to a city which is to be well governed, because he arouses and fosters and strengthens this part of the soul and destroys the reasoning part. Like one who gives a city over into the hands of villains, and destroys the better citizens, so we shall say that the imitative poet likewise implants an evil constitution in the soul of each individual.[28]

In response, Aristotle recommended most forms of dramatic tragedy as an invaluable imitation of the serious problems facing people in real life. He argued that tragedies caused by human ignorance or fallibility (as opposed to those based on stark chance or fate) offered the audience catharsis, the opportunity to find release and provide relief from strong or repressed emotions:

> Tragedy is an imitation of an action that is serious, complete, and of a certain magnitude; in language embellished with each kind of artistic ornament, the several kinds being found in separate parts of the play; in the form of action, not of narrative; through pity and fear effecting the proper purgation of these emotions.[29]

He was not arguing for a strict separation between the moral and the aesthetic. As well as its emotional benefits, Aristotle also considered dramatic poetry to have cognitive value insofar as it deepens our understanding of human experience:

> ... poetry tends to express the universal [...]. By the universal, I mean how a person of a certain type will on occasion speak or act, according to the law of probability or necessity.[30]

This indicates a kinship (rather than a polarity) between poetry and philosophy, since both are concerned with the universal meanings of life.[31] I will explore this link further in Chapter 6.

In 1774, Johann Wolfgang von Goethe published a novel called *The Sorrows of Young Werther*, in which Werther, a sensitive young artist, kills himself with a duelling pistol as the result of an unrequited love affair. This book became an international bestseller and started a phenomenon known as Werther Fever. Much of this was harmless, involving young men dressing up in Werther-style clothing of yellow pants and blue jackets. But there was also a major apprehension across Europe (possibly based more on rumour than fact) about an epidemic of copycat suicides, with young men dressed as Werther shooting themselves with Goethe's novel at their sides. There remains a persistent concern that suicide is socially contagious and that sensationalised or glorified depictions in the media, including literature, may lead to an increase in copycat suicides.[32,33]

But then, in contrast, we also have the Papageno effect, named after the character in Mozart's opera *The Magic Flute*. In one of the opera's final scenes, Papageno decided to hang himself because he has lost his beloved Papagena. He is dissuaded from this drastic course of action by three child spirits, who persuade him to play his magic bells and summon his love back to life again. The argument here is that reports of positive coping in adverse circumstances may have protective effects for suicide prevention.[34]

In this book, I will take the side of Aristotle over Plato, and Papageno over Werther. I will propose (with some caveats) that literary reading has the potential to help people who are living in despair, providing them with sufficient reasons to stay alive. People like Charlie, Frances and Darren, whose stories are based on patients I have met during the past few decades. And people like Leo and Gerard, whose stories I have gathered through their writings. I will support Beth Blum in proposing that literary reading may be a valuable source of self-help.[35] I will argue that engaging with literature, whether in the form of poetry or novels, offers direct help to people who can see little reason to stay alive, for example, in Frances' encounter with the poetry of Gerard Manley Hopkins, and Darren's enthusiasm for Sartre's *Roads to Freedom* trilogy. And people like Matt Haig, who found relief from his depressed isolation through reading Graham Greene's *The Power and the Glory*, the story of a 'whisky priest' traveling through Mexico in the 1930s.

> It is a dark, intense book. But when you are feeling dark and intense these are the only kind of books that can speak to you. Yet there was an optimism too. The possibility of redemption. It is a book about the healing power of love.[36]

I will also argue that literary reading provides powerful indirect help, by strengthening the ability of others – including family doctors like me – to reach out to people contemplating suicide; stretching our imaginations, enhancing our compassion and generating deeper resources within ourselves to enable hope and change.[37] Literature taps into the deep structures of memory and emotion that lie at the heart of our humanity.[38,39] David Kidd and Emanuele Castano, for example, have conducted a series of experiments which show that people assigned to read literary short stories, presenting complex, nuanced characters, subsequently demonstrate greater empathy than people assigned to reading popular genre fiction, presenting more easily understood characters. They propose that reading literary novels increases our empathy because it disrupts our experiences about others' minds, motivations, desires and intentions, forcing us to engage in mind-reading and character construction.[40,41] Such change is welcome and necessary, but is not in itself sufficient. The next step, as Suzanne Keen argues, is to translate our enhanced empathy into real world altruism and effective 'pro-social action'.[42]

There is also an expanding body of research indicating that literary reading, especially in a group setting, can directly improve people's mental health – and hence reduce their propensity to consider suicide.

A few years ago, I was involved with a study of two community-based reading groups, which met weekly for 12 months and read together a wide variety of prose fiction and poetry. There was a clear trend for reduction in depressive symptoms for group participants by the end of the study. We found that reading prose fiction appeared to foster relaxation and calm, while reading poetry encouraged focused concentration. Both literary forms allowed participants to discover new, and rediscover old or forgotten, modes of thought, feeling and experience.

Participants demonstrated an intense absorption that was close to meditation. One man described with surprise, at the close of the first session he attended, how the story they were reading had 'soothed' him 'here', pointing to his forehead. Another participant who during the poetry reading at the start and close of the session had been easily distracted (fidgety in body, eyes and head, and excessively aware of the attention and behaviours of other group members) became stilled as her absorption in the story overcame other claims on her attention.

Expert group facilitation was important in bringing the literature to life, creating an atmosphere of serious attention and holding open key ideas and concerns. And the group members themselves increasingly took the initiative in supporting each other's comments, with discussion at times intense, bursting with simultaneity of thoughts, worlds and realities. In a discussion of Louis McNeice's *Snow*, for example, we find participant A pondering the meaning of the poem and then, with the comment 'Oh strange', shifting away from the text and creating a new world, warm and pleasant.

Participant L immediately joins her in this fantasy world, and mirrors A's syntax as she does so:

A: What's going on and maybe Christmas, maybe just a sudden downfall of snow. Oh, strange. Light the fire, get everything nice and warm.

L: And sit and look out. Out on the world with the snow coming down. [...] More than one thing happens from. You can just imagine yourself being there can't you?

A: Yes.

L: The snow coming down.

A: Yes. Snow us another tangerine [laughs].

L: And the pips.

A: Spitting the pips in the fire.

L: Sitting there in front of the fire, peeling a tangerine.

A: Peeling a tangerine, splitting it up, and the pips in the fire.

L: You can just think of that. You can just imagine that really.

Analysis of the rhythm and intonation of the utterance 'Snow us another tangerine' shows that this playful literary metaphor can also be set to music, reflecting A's exuberant 'singing-out' of the dissolving of boundaries between selves and world.[43]

Further studies of shared reading groups have suggested that they increase people's sense of creativity and purpose in life;[44] and that enhanced literary awareness is related to increased flexibility of internal models of meaning. This heightens subjective awareness of change, and gives a greater capacity to reason about events: all consistent with evidence that relates reading to improved mental well-being.[45]

Robert Piercey suggests that reading can help us to develop our understanding of our lives in three important dimensions.[46] The first is the topic of *selfhood*: this concerns our understanding of what we are, and – in the process – allows us to expand our ideas of what kind of being we are. So, when I am reading George Eliot's *Middlemarch*, I cannot help but put myself in the increasingly unhappy shoes of Tertius Lydgate, as his dreams of a successful modern medical practice disintegrate in the face of a financially and emotionally ruinous marriage. Conversely, when I read the plays of Anton Chekhov or the poetry of William Carlos Williams, I am continually amazed by (and hugely envious of) their abilities to combine such wonderful writing with their work as physicians.

A second set of questions is *ethical*: questions about how to live. These questions may be specific to certain conflicts or dilemmas, or they may deal more generally with what a good life is and how it is best attained.

We will come across such questions many times in the following chapters, not least when sharing in Levin's intense internal debates in *Anna Karenina* on what (if anything) makes life worth living, or when reflecting on Hopkins' call for self-compassion, to *leave comfort root-room*.

Piercey's third set of questions are *ontological*: questions about which things exist and what those things are like. Reading can be a way of reflecting on the nature of things, and on the nature of our relations with things. I have recently been enjoying Robert Macfarlane's *Landmarks*, his exploration of how paying close attention to a particular landscape means we are more likely to behave compassionately towards it; the same is true of attending closely to a particular person, such as myself or my patient. So I would add here that reading is also a way of reflecting on the nature of people, and on the nature of our relations with people.

There is a unique relationship between the literary text and the reader, at any given moment. You and I can read the same poem and we will have different reactions to it. I can read the same poem a week later, and I will have a different reaction to it than I do today. Philip Davis proposes that literary reading involves 'individual acts of triggered contemplation that for some readers have had to become a replacement for religion in the search for human meaning amidst the deeper, darker strata of inner human reality'.[47] While Tolstoy and Hopkins both see their writings are arising from religious belief rather than in replacement of it, those of us who do not share their world-views may still gather invaluable meaning from them.

In her seminal text *Is Literature Healthy?* Josie Billington argues compellingly for the ability of literature to

> 'hold thoughts which humans feel it would almost kill them to contain in themselves...', to acknowledge the deeply unconsolable and to ' "think" reality when ordinary human thought falls short; that a book can have thoughts that humans *cannot* have'.[48]

Andrew Bennett takes this crucial point further, with specific reference to literary works on suicide: Remarking that suicide has 'the unique capacity both to make and to unmake meaning, to offer and remove a life's *sense*', he suggests that

> literature has a particular status since in its engagement with the inadmissible it allows for the possibility of imagining suicide and of feeling empathy towards individuals who undertake it [...]. And it is, we might say, the discourse in which the almost unimaginable grief, anger and guilt that so often follow the suicide of a friend, lover or family member can be construed, figured or imagined.[49]

These perspectives, as we shall see, are of crucial importance when considering how, for example, reading about the final minutes of Anna Karenina's life enables us to entertain (and survive) otherwise unimaginably distressing thoughts and emotions.

Literary reading enables us to give voice to thoughts and experiences that would otherwise be too difficult to contemplate. It offers us safe psychological distance, partly because it is 'other' and partly because we can exercise control and agency over it: we can choose to engage with the text, or we can choose to close it or throw it away. If we can read it, we can more readily endure it. If we can come face to face with the darkest elements of life, we can look them squarely in the eye, and refuse to be defeated.

Themes of This Book

In Chapter 2, I consider theories designed to explain why people may decide not to stay alive. I begin with an overview of early modern theories of suicidal ideas and behaviour, starting with Durkheim's sociological perspectives on *anomie* and normlessness, linking back in time to Marx on alienation. I note Freud's psychoanalytic understanding of mourning and melancholia, and recent sociobiological theories of altruistic suicide. I then provide a sympathetic critique of contemporary explanations, drawing on sociological, psychological and anthropological perspectives. I conclude with reflections on how these perspectives may inform our understanding and interpretation of suicidal ideas and actions in literary texts.

In Chapter 3, I examine how the dilemma of existence plays out in Leo Tolstoy's *Anna Karenina*. Anna's suicide is the most dramatic encounter with death in the novel, but it is far from the only one. Kitty, Vronsky and Levin (Tolstoy's alter-ego) also find themselves uncertain about whether – or why – to stay alive. I use the psychosocial models from Chapter 2 as starting points to explore the reasons for their differing outcomes. I reflect on how Tolstoy's literary expression of profound existential tensions, in *Anna Karenina* and elsewhere, inform my understanding of the life experiences of Charlie.

Building on my earlier exploration of Gerard Manley Hopkins' poetry, in Chapter 4, I undertake a detailed analysis of the turmoil and despair he expresses, and works through, in his so-called terrible sonnets. Created during a deeply unhappy period of his life while employed as a Classics professor in University College Dublin, these six poems arise from 'a languishment of body and mind'. Yet these sonnets also give their readers, including me and Frances, glimpses of his unimpeachable honesty, of the legitimacy of distress, and a sense of connection, of shared experience. They encourage the ability to observe our emotions rather than be overwhelmed by them, the determination to survive come what may, and the flowering of self-compassion.

In Chapter 5, I move the chronological dial forwards and backwards to consider more generally how literary and poetic texts confront the dilemma of existence in the face of grief and loss, and how literary readings can offer points of transformation, new conversations with patients, with loved ones and ourselves. We can find help in more or less expected sources, from an ancient Egyptian papyrus to twenty-first-century comedic fiction. With Al Alvarez, we may acknowledge that suicide offers no resolution or salvation, and is (most likely) merely the end of experience. We may be persuaded by Stevie Smith that death is to be earned, not grasped before its time, and find resolve in the ways in which contemporary poets and writers confront the seriousness of living through troubled times. We may come to realise that it is possible not only to survive but even to thrive, despite our own close encounters with suicide or the inexplicable death of someone we have loved.

In Chapter 6, I examine how the existential question, whether it is better to be or not to be, remains prominent not only in *Hamlet* but also in moral philosophy. Pessimistic philosophers may lead us towards alarming conclusions, unless their views are tempered by compassion. I have previously proposed a concept of the self, deriving from two interacting components of coherence and engagement. Reviewing these arguments in the context of suicide, and with the benefit of the insights gained from my encounters with Tolstoy and Hopkins, I consider how our sense of coherence, our desire to persevere in our own being, may become overwhelmed; and propose that engagement – whether communal, spiritual or political – is critical to the existential preservation of the self, enabling us to recover or create reasons to be. I work through this proposition, with help from my interactions with Darren.

In the final chapter, I review and reflect on lessons learned from my encounters with Tolstoy and Hopkins and other literary texts, in terms of the ways in which we address ideas of suicide, and how they can inform our therapeutic encounters. I note how these approaches may equally be applied to other visual and performing arts, including painting, sculpture and music. I consider their potential impact on commonly used preventative approaches, now extended to include the possibility – and reality – of survival, hope and flourishing. I explore ways in which I as a family doctor, and others in caring positions may act as catalysts or reagents, or simply bear witness, to the processes of transformation away from death and towards life.

Perspectives

My writing emerges from my own personal background, and in the context of my particular clinical practice. It addresses my own life, and the lives of the patients I see, so often troubled by poverty and precarity. It is authentic, but necessarily limited.

The literary and scientific texts I engage with are focused primarily on white, western subjects, and almost all use English as their first language. These cultural factors inevitably restrict the boundaries of my thoughts and enquiries. I do not consider myself competent to discuss, for example, the Japanese novels of Yukio Mishima, with their assertion of the unity of beauty, eroticism and death. Nor do I have the personal or cultural background to do justice to the rich complexity of suicide narratives explored by writers of African descent such as Toni Morrison and Ntozake Shange.

Other stories, other perspectives, are both possible and necessary. I hope that readers will engage with me and share their own understandings and experiences. Together we can create a richer collection of literary resources to enable people confronting the dilemma of their existence to stay alive.

It is important to acknowledge that the topic of this book and the narratives within it, whether real or fictive, may be deeply troubling at a personal level. Writing about them has at times been challenging for me. I am aware that reading about them may be distressing for readers too, not least if a particular story or description triggers personal memories or emotional reactions. If it does, I urge you to take your time, put the book to one side for a while, and share your concerns with somebody you trust.

Notes

1 Leo Tolstoy, *A Confession and Other Religious Writings*, trans. Jane Kentish (London: Penguin Book, 1987), 33.

2 Gerard Manley Hopkins, 'Letter to Robert Bridges', *Poems and Prose of Gerard Manley Hopkins*, ed. William Gardner (London: Penguin Books, 1968), 17 May 1885, 202.

3 Diego De Leo et al., 'Definitions of Suicidal Behavior: Lessons Learned from the WHO/EURO Multicentre Study'. *Crisis* 27, no. 1 (2006): 4–15.

4 Seena Fazel and Bo Runeson, 'Suicide'. *New England Journal of Medicine* 382, no. 3 (2020): 266–74.

5 World Health Organisation, 'Suicide', 17 June 2021. Accessed 18 August 2021. https://www.who.int/news-room/fact-sheets/detail/suicide.

6 Julie Cerel et al., 'How Many People Are Exposed to Suicide? Not Six'. *Suicide and Life Threatening Behavior* 49, no. 2 (2019): 529–34.

7 Sally McManus et al., eds. *Mental Health and Wellbeing in England: Adult Psychiatric Morbidity Survey 2014* (Leeds: NHS Digital, 2016), 301.

8 Matthew Nock et al., 'Cross-National Prevalence and Risk Factors for Suicidal Ideation, Plans and Attempts'. *British Journal of Psychiatry* 192, no. 2 (2008): 98–105.

9 Kathryn Piscopo et al., 'Suicidal Thoughts and Behavior among Adults: Results from the 2015 National Survey on Drug Use and Health'. September 2016. Accessed 18 August 2021. https://www.samhsa.gov/data/sites/default/files/NSDUH-DR-FFR3-2015/NSDUH-DR-FFR3-2015.htm#topofpage.

10 Daisy Fancourt et al., 'COVID-19 Social Study. Results Release 7', 6 May 2020. Accessed 18 August 2021. https://www.covidsocialstudy.org/results.

11 Faraz Mughal et al., 'Role of the GP in the Management of Patients with Self-Harm Behaviour: A Systematic Review'. *British Journal of General Practice* 70, no. 694 (2020): e364–e373.

12 Carl May et al., 'Experiences of Long-Term Life-Limiting Conditions among Patients and Carers: What Can We Learn from a Meta-Review of Systematic Reviews of Qualitative Studies of Chronic Heart Failure, Chronic Obstructive Pulmonary Disease and Chronic Kidney Disease?' *BMJ Open* 6, no. 10 (2016): e011694.

13 Amy Chandler et al., 'The Social Life of Self-Harm in General Practice'. *Social Theory and Health* 18, no. 3 (2020): 240–56.

14 Tommaso Dazzi et al., 'Does Asking about Suicide and Related Behaviours Induce Suicidal Ideation? What Is the Evidence?' *Psychological Medicine* 44, no. 16 (2014): 3361–63.

15 Lindsey Sinclair and Richard Leach, 'Exploring Thoughts of Suicide', *British Medical Journal* 356 (2017): j1128.

16 Priyanka Dube et al., 'The p4 Screener: Evaluation of a Brief Measure for Assessing Potential Suicide Risk in 2 Randomized Effectiveness Trials of Primary Care and Oncology Patients'. *The Primary Care Companion to the Journal of Clinical Psychiatry* 12, no. 6 (2010): PCC.10m00978.

17 Chani Nuij et al., 'Safety-Planning Type Interventions for Suicide Prevention: Meta-Analysis'. *British Journal of Psychiatry* 219, no. 2 (2021): 419–26.

18 Verity Wainwright et al., 'Experiences of Support from Primary Care and Perceived Needs of Parents Bereaved by Suicide: A Qualitative study'. *British Journal of General Practice* 70, no. 691 (2020): e102–e110.

19 Alys Cole-King and Siobhan O'Neill, 'Suicide Prevention', in *Primary Care Mental Health*, 2nd edition, ed. Linda Gask et al. (Cambridge: Cambridge University Press, 2018), 103–24.

20 Geraldine Strathdee et al., 'Risk Assessment and Management of Suicidality in Primary Care Mental Health', in *Companion to Primary Care Mental Health*, ed. Gabriel Ivbijaro (London: Radcliffe, 2012), 178–203.

21 World Health Organisation, *mhGAP Intervention Guide 2.0*. (Geneva: WHO, 2016), 131–40. Accessed 7 January 2021. https://www.who.int/publications/i/item/mhgap-intervention-guide---version-2.0.

22 World Health Organisation, *Live Life: Implementation Guide for Suicide Prevention in Countries* (WHO: Geneva, 2021). Accessed 12 August 2021. https://www.who.int/publications/i/item/9789240026629.

23 Matt Haig, *Reasons to Stay Alive* (London: Canongate, 2015).

24 Rory O'Connor, *When It Is Darkest: Why People Die by Suicide and What We Can Do to Prevent It* (London: Penguin, 2021).

25 Christopher Dowrick, *Beyond Depression*, 2nd edition (Oxford: Oxford University Press, 2009).

26 Christopher Dowrick, 'Comfort in a Whirlwind: Literature and Distress in General Practice', in *Reading and Mental Health*, ed. Josie Billington (Cham: Palgrave Macmillan, 2019), 15–30.

27 Friedrich Nietzsche, *The Birth of Tragedy*, trans. Clifton Padiman (Mineola, NY: Dover Publications, 1995).

28 Plato, *The Republic*, trans. Alexander Lindsay (London: Dent, Everyman Books, 1935): book 10, section 605, 308–9.

29 Aristotle, *Poetics*, trans. Samuel Butcher (Project Gutenberg eBook, 2013) Book VI. Accessed 18 April 2021. https://www.gutenberg.org/files/1974/1974-h/1974-h. htm#link2H_4_0008.

30 Aristotle, ibid. Book IX.

31 Stephen Halliwell, 'Plato and Aristotle on the Denial of Tragedy', *Proceedings of the Cambridge Philological Society* 210, no. 30 (1984): 49–71.

32 Anna Mueller and Seth Abrutyn, 'Suicidal Disclosures among Friends: Using Social Network Data to Understand Suicide Contagion'. *Journal of Health and Social Behaviour* 56, no. 1 (2015): 131–48.

33 Thomas Niederkrotenthaler et al., 'Association between Suicide Reporting in the Media and Suicide: Systematic Review and Meta-Analysis'. *British Medical Journal*, 368 (2020): m575.

34 Thomas Niederkrotenthaler et al., 'Role of Media Reports in Completed and Prevented Suicide: Werther v. Papageno Effects'. *British Journal of Psychiatry* 197, no. 3 (2010): 234–43.

35 Beth Blum, *The Self-Help Compulsion: Searching for Advice in Modern Literature* (New York: Columbia University Press, 2020).

36 Matt Haig, *Reasons to Stay Alive*, 135.

37 Robert Downie, *The Healing Arts* (Oxford: Oxford University Press, 1994).

38 Christopher Comer and Asley Taggart, *Brain, Mind and the Narrative Imagination* (London: Bloomsbury, 2021).

39 Angus Fletcher, *Wonderworks: Literary Invention and the Science of Stories* (New York: Simon & Schuster, 2021).

40 David Kidd and Emanuele Castano, 'Reading Literary Fiction Improves Theory of Mind'. *Science* 342, no. 6156 (2013): 377–80.

41 David Kidd and Emanuele Castano, 'Reading Literary Fiction Can Improve Theory of Mind'. *Nature Human Behaviour* 2 (2018): 604.

42 Suzanne Keen, *Empathy and the Novel* (Oxford: Oxford University Press, 2007).

43 Christopher Dowrick et al., 'Get into Reading as an Intervention for Common Mental Health Problems: Exploring Catalysts for Change'. *Medical Humanities*, 38, no. 1 (2012): 15–20.

44 Eleanor Longden et al., 'Shared Reading: Assessing the Intrinsic Value of a Literature-Based Health Intervention'. *Medical Humanities* 41, no. 2 (2015): 113–20.

45 Noreen O'Sullivan et al., ' "Shall I Compare Thee": The Neural Basis of Literary Awareness, and Its Benefits to Cognition'. *Cortex*, 73 (2015): 144–57.

46 Robert Piercey, *Reading as Philosophical Practice* (London/New York: Anthem Press, 2021).

47 Phil Davis, *Reading for Life* (Oxford: Oxford University Press, 2020), 5.

48 Josie Billington, *Is Literature Healthy?* (Oxford: Oxford University Press, 2016), 31, 44.

49 Andrew Bennett, *Suicide Century: Literature and Suicide from James Joyce to David Foster Wallace* (Cambridge: Cambridge University Press, 2017), 20.

Chapter 2

THWARTED BELONGINGNESS

One cannot long remain so absorbed in contemplation of emptiness without being increasingly attracted to it. In vain one bestows on it the name of infinity; this does not change its nature. When one feels such pleasure in non-existence, one's inclination can be completely satisfied only by completely ceasing to exist.[1]

Before exploring how literary reading can help people in despair decide to stay alive, in this chapter, I am going to review contemporary theories of suicidal behaviour, drawing mainly on ideas from social psychology and cultural anthropology. I believe this will be helpful, initially, in enabling better understanding of how suicidal ideas are presented in literary texts. And then, later in the book, I will suggest ways in which literary reading can usefully inform, modify and extend these theories.

Anomie and Alienation

Sociological perspectives probably start with Emile Durkheim's *Suicide*, published in Paris in 1897.[2] Durkheim took the view, radical in his day, that suicide was not the result of deep moral failure, nor simply an individual's response to difficult life circumstances. Instead, it should be understood as a *social* fact, that is to say something that is external to, and imposed upon, individual actors. He drew attention to the effects of imbalance between social regulation and social integration. Social regulation is understood as the normative or moral demands placed on the individual that come with membership in a group, while social integration refers to the extent of social relations binding a person or a group to others, such that they are exposed to the moral demands of the group. On this basis he proposed four different types of suicide.

Egotistic suicide reflects a sense of not belonging, of having no stake in a community and results from a lack of social integration.

This is connected with a general state of extreme depression and exaggerated sadness, causing the patient no longer to realize sanely the bonds which connect him with people and things about him. Pleasures no longer attract.[3]

Durkheim argued that detachment, or what he called 'excessive individuation', meant people had little social support or guidance. He found that suicide was more common amongst unmarried men, who had few social connections. Linking back to the stories I presented in Chapter 1, this is the position Charlie finds herself in, critically ill with cancer, cut off from contact with her family, especially her beloved granddaughter, and socially isolated in the midst of the COVID-19 pandemic. As we shall see in Chapter 4, it also applies to Gerard Manley Hopkins, adrift from family and friends in the (to him) alien environment of Ireland.

Altruistic suicide, with too much social integration, reflects a sense of being overwhelmed by a group's goals and beliefs. This is more common in societies where individual needs are seen as less important than society's needs as a whole. Durkheim saw military service as an example of this, where the individual soldier is expected to risk his own death on behalf of society. We have Captain Laurence Oates, aware that the gangrene and frostbite from which he was suffering was compromising his three companions' chances of survival, walking out of their tent into a blizzard in the hope of preserving the lives of his fellow explorers on the Terra Nova Expedition of Antarctica in 1912. According to expedition leader Robert Scott's diary, Oates' last words were 'I am just going outside. I may be some time'.[4] This line of argument has also been taken up by evolutionary biologists, who suggest an instinct towards self-sacrifice for the good of surviving relatives, either because those relatives will be rescued from their own death or because they will benefit richly from the resources that are thus freed up. The survivors will in turn pass on the sacrificial victim's genes.[5] In literature, for example, we find Maggie O'Farrell's Hamnet giving up his own life to save his twin sister Judith from bubonic plague:[6] I will explore this story further in Chapter 5.

Anomic suicide, with too little social regulation, reflects a sense of aimlessness and despair, as we can see in the quotation on the 'contemplation of emptiness' at the beginning of this chapter. Durkheim related this to dramatic social or economic upheaval, for example, periods of rapid mass economic migration from rural to urban areas, when it becomes impossible for the individual to predict what life has or should have to offer. This was a major problem in late nineteenth-century France, as it is in many low- and middle-income countries today – and for the millions forced to leave their known worlds in the face of political and humanitarian disaster.

Fatalistic suicide, with too much social regulation, reflects a life is overshadowed by excessive discipline, when one has no choice but to follow the same routine day after day. Durkheim suggested that prisoners might prefer to die than to live in a prison with constant abuse and excessive regulation. This is a factor in the high rates of suicide amongst young married women in rural China who have low social status, and limited freedom when faced with forbidding cultural expectations and negative social relations.[7] My patient Frances displays some of these characteristics, although much of her excessive discipline has, over the years, become self-imposed.

Durkheim's writings on anomie link back to Karl Marx's theories of alienation: of man as a sensuous, suffering and passionate being[8] with a profound sense of social dislocation: alienated from his work since he plays no part in deciding what to do or how to do it, alienated from his own products since he has no control over what he makes or what becomes of it afterwards, and alienated from his fellow men, since competition renders most forms of cooperation impossible:[9]

> The savage in his cave – a natural element which freely offers itself for his use and protection – feels himself no more a stranger, or rather feels himself to be just as much at home as a fish in water. But the cellar-dwelling of the poor man is a hostile dwelling, 'an alien, restraining power which only gives itself up to him in so far as he gives up to it his blood and sweat' – a dwelling which he cannot look upon as his own home where he might at last exclaim, 'here I am at home', but where instead he finds himself in someone else's house, in the house of a stranger who daily lies in wait for him and throws him out if he does not pay his rent.[10]

Melancholia and Thanatos

Meanwhile in Vienna, Sigmund Freud was considering how intense internal psychological conflicts generate thoughts of suicide.

In his early writings on how the unconscious mind affects much of our everyday life, he observed that our tendency towards self-destruction is much more common than we generally wish to believe:

> Anyone who believes in the occurrence of half-intentional self-*injury [...]* will be prepared to assume that in addition to consciously intentional suicide there is such a thing as half-intentional self-*destruction* (self-destruction with an unconscious intention), capable of making skilful use of a threat to life and of disguising it as a chance mishap. There is no need to think such self-destruction rare.[11]

Then in 1917, in his seminal paper on mourning and melancholia, he developed his theories more formally, proposing that ideas of suicide occur when hostility towards another person is turned inwards on oneself; in other words, that hate has a suicide-inducing effect. Suicide can happen when the object to which one is attached and which one is unable to let go (for example, a parent or partner who has died), is also the target of one's hostility, anger, rage and aggression.

> So we find the key to the clinical picture: we perceive that the self-reproaches are reproaches against a loved object which have been shifted away from it on to the patient's own ego.[12]

Killing oneself in these circumstances, according to Freud, is an aggressive act. Suicidal thoughts themselves are a fantasy of trying to control an overwhelming process, or even of making someone else pay for something they did. He might, for example, interpret Leo Tolstoy's suicidal impulses as repressed anger towards his admired elder brother dying of tuberculosis, or his father, or (perhaps most significantly) his mother for leaving him when he was only two.

Later in his life, following the devastation of the first world war and the consequent social and political instability across Europe, Freud expanded his focus from the personal to the societal. In his final and most dramatic formulation of human instincts, he proposed that human beings have a fundamentally aggressive nature; with the incessant conflict between love and death – *eros* and *thanatos* – as the basis of civilisation and its discontents:

> [...] men are not gentle creatures who want to be loved, and who at the most can defend themselves if they are attacked; they are on the contrary, creatures amongst whose instinctual endowments are to be reckoned a powerful share of aggressiveness. As a result their neighbour is for them [...] someone who tempts them to satisfy their aggressiveness on him, to exploit his capacity for work without compensation, to use him sexually without his consent, to humiliate him, to cause him pain, to torture and to kill him. *Homo homini lupus* [...]
>
> This aggressive instinct is the derivative and the main representative of the death instinct which we have found alongside of Eros and which shares world domination with it. And now, I think, the meaning of the evolution of civilization is no longer obscure to us. It must represent the struggle between Eros and Death, between the instinct of life and the instinct of destruction, as it works itself out in the human species. And it is this battle of the giants that our nursemaids try to appease with their lullaby about Heaven.[13]

Robert Roland Smith argues that Freud's death drive is primarily an unconscious desire for inertia, and as such is closer to preservation than to annihilation. He suggests that suicide falls 'outside the bailiwick of the death-drive'.[14] However, it seems to me (and to Al Alvarez, as we shall see in Chapter 5) that we can all too easily turn this battle of the giants, these aggressive impulses, this death instinct, back upon ourselves.

Social Roots of Suicide

The current understandings of suicidal thoughts and actions that I find most persuasive combine social, psychological and anthropological elements.

Anna Mueller and Seth Abrutyn have recently developed a seminal body of work, generating important insights into the mechanisms underpinning Durkheim's observations of the impact of an individual's membership of a particular group or category. They draw our attention to the ways in which our identities, and the emotional attachment we have to those identities, help to make sense of why certain structures and cultures may be harmful or protective. In doing so, they bridge the gap between external social facts and internal individual actions and behaviours.

Mueller and Abrutyn identify four key aspects of identity and emotion.[15] First, people whose identity is embedded in a relationship, a group or broader social system will feel higher levels of commitment to that identity; their commitment will depend on both the intimate, emotional aspects and the extent of their social ties. Second, when commitment to an identity is high, the person will also be emotionally attached to the bond itself. Third, the more committed an individual is to a particular identity, and attached to a particular bond, the more influence other members of their group have on their feelings, thoughts, and actions. Fourth, where fewer alternative identities and bonds exist, cultural regulation will be at its most powerful, because a continued sense of commitment and attachment is more desirable than the experience of exclusion and isolation.

> Identity matters, then to suicide and mental health, because it is one prominent pathway through which the external social world comes to matter to perceptions of self. Our identity renders painful the possibility of exclusion, rejection, and isolation from cherished social groups, not simply because we feel lonely, but because a part of our self can be damaged or lost through these social experiences.[16]

Failure, or fear of failure, lead to shame, a painful social emotion indicating that the person believes others to judge them as deficient. Negative social emotions like shame are signals that our essential social connections are in danger, dissolving or indeed already lost. In cultures with strong traditions of male norms, such as contemporary Ghana, failure to meet masculine expectation is closely tied to suicide as a way of restoring honour.[17] I will show in Chapter 3 how this scenario plays out in the case of Count Vronsky, a member of the elite army officer corps in late nineteenth-century Russia.

We can also see the continuing influence of Durkheim through the lens of Robert Merton's strain theory, which proposes that society puts pressure on individuals to achieve socially accepted goals despite not having the means to do so.[18] Although strain theory has been applied most commonly to analysis of criminality, it is also relevant to suicidal behaviour, focusing on strains or pressures coming from contradictory directions that push a person towards despair.

Jie Zhang observes that suicide is usually preceded by some psychological strains. A strain is not simply psychological pressure or stress, but develops in the presence of two or more conflicting pressures or variables: 'Similar to the formation of cognitive dissonance, but more serious and detrimental than cognitive dissonance, a strain pulls or pushes an individual in different directions so as to make them frustrated, upset, angry or even to feel pain'.[19]

Zhang identifies four sources of strain which can lead to suicide. First is strain from differential values, from 'two competing personal beliefs internalized in the person's value system'; for example, the strain amongst second-generation immigrants in the United States who have to abide by the ethnic culture rules of their family while adapting to American culture with peers and school; or (as we shall see in Chapter 5) the strain of Paul Sheringham, torn between loving Jane Fairchild, a domestic servant, and his family's expectation that he will marry within his own class. Second is strain from the discrepancy between aspiration and reality, between one's splendid ideal or goal and the circumstances that stand in the way of one's achieving it; for example, a young woman in rural China seeking equal opportunity in a community with conservative Confucian gender values;[20] or Anna Karenina wishing to live together with her lover Vronsky and with her son Sergei, in a society where that is a legal impossibility. Third is the strain arising from relative deprivation, where the conflicting social facts are 'one's own miserable life and the perceived wealth of comparative others'; for example, in an economically polarised society where rich and poor live close to each other. And the fourth type of strain he terms 'deficient coping', arising from a lack of coping skills in the face of a crisis, for example, a boy being bullied in high school who does not know how to deal with the situation; or a woman (like Charlie) abused by her partner in the absence of support from other family members.

The pathway from strain to suicidal ideas and actions is supported by research studies in China.[21,22] It can be moderated by social and psychological factors, attitudes and beliefs, including religion. In one study of more than a thousand employees in Bejing, Zhang and his team found that the impact of strain on suicidality was moderated and decreased by the presence of social support.[23]

Belonging and Burden

Thomas Joiner's Interpersonal Theory (IPT) proposes that the most dangerous form of suicidal desire, leading to lethal or near-lethal suicidal attempts, is caused by the simultaneous presence of two experiences or ideas – thwarted belongingness and perceived burdensomeness – when combined with a capability for acting on the desire[24] (see Figure 2.1).[25]

We humans are social beings: we have a deeply felt need to belong, to be accepted, appreciated and loved by others. Since social isolation is one of the strongest and most reliable predictors of suicidal ideation, IPT proposes that 'social connectedness variables are associated with suicide because they are observable indicators that a fundamental human psychological need is unmet'. This is the need which Joiner calls *thwarted belongingness.*

Thwarted belongingness has two main elements: loneliness, a feeling of disconnectedness, an unpleasant emotional response to perceived isolation, the perception of being alone and isolated; and the absence of reciprocally caring relationships, the lack of another living being to share the ups and downs of life with. It is not necessarily a permanent state of affairs; it can be influenced by external factors, such as the number of people in your social network, and also by internal factors, such as your current emotional state. If you are feeling low in mood and depressed, you are more likely to feel

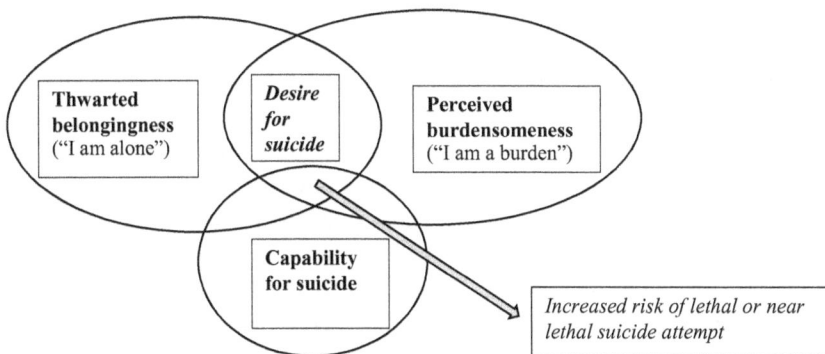

Figure 2.1 Interpersonal theory of suicide model.

thwarted by a lack of belonging to anything or anyone. Joiner and colleagues further propose that suicidal ideas are more likely to emerge if a sense of thwarted belongingness goes on for a long time, is prolonged and intractable; and if meaningful and mutually supportive connections are completely or permanently absent, for example, for a prisoner in solitary confinement. So, on the other hand, if we are fortunate enough to be in positive long-term relationships, have children and access to a wide circle of friends, we are much more likely to want to stay alive.

Perceived burdensomeness, the idea that I am a burden, a weight, a drain on or a nuisance to other people, is most commonly linked to personal experiences of family conflict, unemployment or physical illness. In any of these circumstances, a person may come to believe that they are a liability to others, develop a sense of self-dislike or even self-hatred, and arrive at the apparently logical conclusion that the world would be better off without them. For example, a psychological autopsy conducted on people with terminal cancer who died by suicide showed that self-perceptions of being a burden on others was a key characteristic which contributed to a person's desire for suicide.[26]

These two constructs are more likely to co-exist if someone is presently suffering from a mental disorder such as depression or social anxiety, and if they have experienced adverse childhood events, such as physical or verbal violence, sexual abuse, and physical or emotional neglect.[27]

IPT further suggests that the *capability for suicide*, our willingness not just to contemplate but actually to engage in suicidal behaviour, emerges in response to repeated exposure to physically pain and fear inducing experiences. Although we humans are biologically predisposed to fear suicide, and have an inbuilt desire to survive, it is possible to reduce this fear and become more tolerant of pain: 'through repeated practice, what was originally a painful and/or fear-inducing experience (i.e., self-injury) may become less frightening as well as a source of emotional relief'. So, people who have been exposed to physical abuse or other adverse experiences in childhood or experienced intimate partner violence as adults, members of the armed forces who have had direct experience of combat, or those who have made previous self-harm or suicide attempts:[28] all of these people will be more used to both fear and pain, and as a result become more able to tolerate them.[29]

However, this is not a straightforward cause-and-effect process. For example, while being a member of the military may increase a soldier's capability to engage in suicidal behaviour, the opportunity to form close interpersonal bonds may increase their social connections and hence reduce their sense of thwarted belongingness: as a result, they may be less likely to wish to take self-harming actions.[30]

The IPT of suicide has been subjected to rigorous testing, and there is emerging evidence of its validity. Loneliness is a significant predictor of both suicidal ideation and behaviour, especially amongst women, teenagers and older people.[31] A major systematic review and meta-analysis of studies involving almost 60,000 participants, many of whom were college students and current or past members of the armed forces, came to two main conclusions: that the interaction between thwarted belongingness and perceived burdensomeness was significantly associated with suicidal ideation; and that the interaction between thwarted belongingness, perceived burdensomeness, and capability for suicide was significantly related to a greater number of prior suicide attempts.

Carol Chu and colleagues note that increasing one's capability to engage in suicide can have positive as well as negative effects: 'depending on the context, it can have admirable qualities (e.g., resolve, endurance) as well as ones that can be sad, savage, and lethal (e.g., a violent suicide attempt)'.[32] Several patients have told me that knowing they could end their lives whenever they choose does, paradoxically, give them the ability to endure hard times. As a family doctor I do find it a worrying thought, that they may have a secret stash of sleeping pills somewhere; but it does seem to help some people keep going.

So my patient Darren, whom I introduced at the beginning of the previous chapter, appears to me to be at quite a high risk of suicide. His sense of belongingness, already limited because he has little contact with his family, is further thwarted by the strains in his relationship with his partner, and by the death of his much-loved dog. He has been unemployed for several years, and parting company with his band means he has little chance of changing that just now: a lot of the time he sees himself as a burden to others, 'just a waste of space'. And he has clear capability to engage in suicidal behaviour, given his experience of abuse as a child, his fights with friends, nightclub doormen and police and – especially, his frequent acts of self-harm with razors.

Defeat and Entrapment

Building on Joiner's work, Rory O'Connor and Olivia Kirtley propose an Integrated Motivational-Volitional (IMV) model of suicidal behaviour, in which perceptions of defeat and entrapment drive the emergence of suicidal ideation.[33] A group of factors which they call volitional moderators, including fearlessness about death, increased pain tolerance and mental imagery, then govern the transition from suicidal ideation to suicidal behaviour. The IMV model has three sections, as we can see in Figure 2.2.[34]

Starting with the *pre-motivational phase*, the IMV model describes the background factors and events which may trigger the emergence of

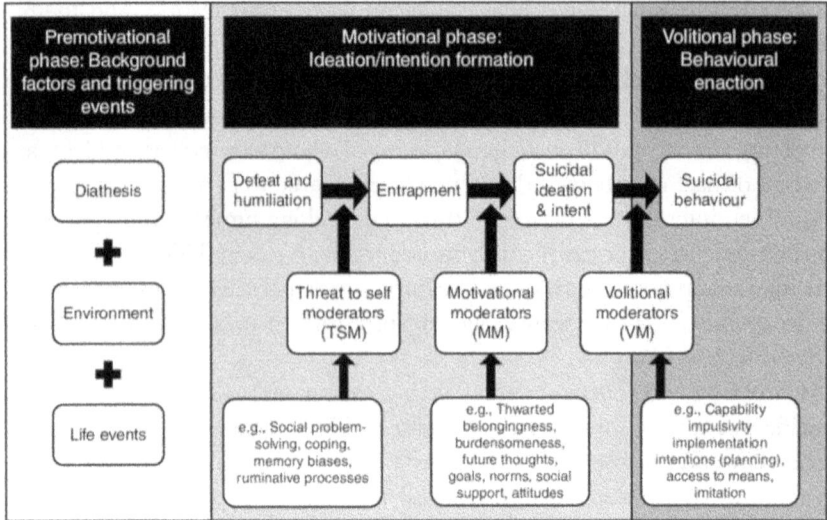

Figure 2.2 Integrated motivational-volitional model of suicidal behaviour.

suicidal ideas and behaviours. It recognises that we may have personal, individual vulnerabilities which increase our risk of developing suicidal ideas in the presence of particular stressful environments and events. So, for example, a tendency to perfectionism, the belief that we have to be successful and high achievers, is more likely to make us downcast and perceive ourselves as failures when we find ourselves trapped in poverty or exposed to persistent racial harassment, or when we find unexpected obstacles in our way, such as failure to pass a necessary academic examination, or the emergence of a new and potentially fatal viral infection.

The model then considers factors leading to the emergence of suicidal ideation in the *motivational phase*. Central to this phase of the IMV model is the idea that a sense of *defeat* and *entrapment* can lead to the emergence of suicidal ideation. O'Connor and Kirtley explain how these elements are drawn from a concept known as 'arrested flight', which was adopted from evolutionary psychology and originally used to explain behavioural states observed in individuals with depression. Arrested flight describes the experience of feeling as though one has been brought down (defeated) and has no prospect of escape or rescue (entrapment).[35] These concepts characterize well the 'tunnel vision' often observed in individuals experiencing suicidal distress, whereby suicide becomes the only perceived escape route.[36]

They note that humiliation also features within this theory, but that less attention has been paid to it than to defeat and entrapment. They propose that the link between defeat and entrapment may be increased by a tendency to ruminate on one's life difficulties, and mitigated by a belief in one's ability to solve social problems. They agree with Joiner that thwarted belongingness and perceived burdensomeness are important in moving from a sense of entrapment to generating suicidal ideas sense of defeat and entrapment; but they also note that depleted resilience – an inability to 'bounce back' when life becomes hard – has a part to play in taking this crucial next step.

Finally, the IMV model describes the factors involved in someone making the transition from suicidal ideation to attempting death by suicide, in the volitional phase.[37] Again, O'Connor and colleagues agree with Joiner's that fearlessness about death and increased physical pain tolerance are important stepping stones from contemplating suicide to acting on it. However, they believe that there are other factors in play here. They note that exposure to the suicidal behaviour of others, especially family and friends, increases the likelihood that someone will attempt to kill themselves when they encounter a stressful event, and that glamourising suicide on film, television or social media (social contagion, the so-called Werther Effect that I noted in Chapter 1) may also do so.[38] Non-fictional presentations of celebrities' suicides in newspapers and on television news appear to have the biggest influence on subsequent risk of suicide.[39] Access to the means to end one's life is important, as is mental imagery of suicide: O'Connor and Kirtley suggest that 'mental imagery increases the likelihood of enactment as it acts as a form of cognitive rehearsal for the behaviour'.

As with IPT, there is evidence emerging to support the IMV model of suicide. The most valuable sources of evidence are prospective studies, where predictions about ideas and behaviours are tested into the future, rather than by reviewing past events, thus reducing the likelihood of false or misleading inferences and associations. In a study of 70 patients who had been admitted to hospital following a suicide attempt, a sense of entrapment was an independent predictor of readmission to hospital for self-harm within the next four years.[40] Three studies, one of people with bipolar disorder and the other two of adults living in the community, have found evidence that perceived burdensomeness and a sense of entrapment are related to a sense of defeat and hence, to the emergence or persistence of suicidal ideation.[41,42,43] One study, involving over 3,500 young adults in Scotland has assessed how the ITP and IMV models might work together. It found support for these models in combination, as core factors from each model – internal entrapment from the IMV model and perceived burdensomeness from the IPT model – were strongly related to suicide ideation in this group of people.[44]

Using the IMV model as a guide, Charlie's risk of suicide is high. In her background, or pre-motivational phase, she has a long history of vulnerability in the form of psychological and racial harassment from her partner, and this is aggravated by the severity of her current physical health problems. She feels persistently humiliated by him, and indeed by the ways in which her children tend to take his side. Although she is no longer ostensibly trapped in her relationship with him, since moving out of the family home, she finds it very hard to disengage from him emotionally; her attempts to re-establish some degree of communication with her family usually end in defeat, a problem exacerbated by the social distancing requirements of the pandemic. Her resilience is severely depleted. And she is already in the volitional stage, using alcohol to numb her senses and having taken at least two overdoses of painkillers and antidepressants in recent months.

Sense of Safety

My next contemporary perspective is Johanna Lynch's concept of *sense of safety*. Arising from a transdisciplinary understanding of attachment and trauma-informed approaches, this concept is based on two simple but powerful questions: what threatens people and where (if anywhere) do we feel safe? It offers invaluable insights into the enormously wide range of threats that we may face, from our environment, through our extended and intimate social relationships, to our physical and psychic experiences, and our inner sense of self, meaning and spirit[45], as summarised in Figure 2.3.[46]

Contextual or environmental threats may arise from the impact of climate change and consequent natural disasters including famine, floods (like those currently causing havoc in northern Europe) or fires (such as those raging in Siberia as I write), or from political conflicts, such as the civil wars in Syria and Yemen and the implosion of civil society in Venezuela. For example, the climate crisis has a detrimental impact on the mental health and wellbeing of children and young people, with a range of psychological effects including an increase in suicidal thinking.[47] Threats to our social climate, in our local or wider communities, are heightened for members of ethnic minorities,[48,49] for people who are homeless and do not have a safe place to sleep,[50] and for women in public spaces.[51] Social threats may be more personal, as they are for Darren in his attempts to seek justice from benefits agencies. Relational threats are all too common, whether from the intimate partner violence perpetrated over many years on Charlie; or from the opposite, the persistent sense of loneliness and isolation that is Frances' daily experience.

Our bodies may be under threat from assault (as for Charlie) from infections, such as COVID-19, from acute diseases such as coronary infarction or pulmonary embolism, or from chronic illnesses such as diabetes or rheumatoid disease. Our inner experiences – our 'thoughts, attention, memories, perceptions, sense, intuition, mood states and self-talk' may (like Frances)

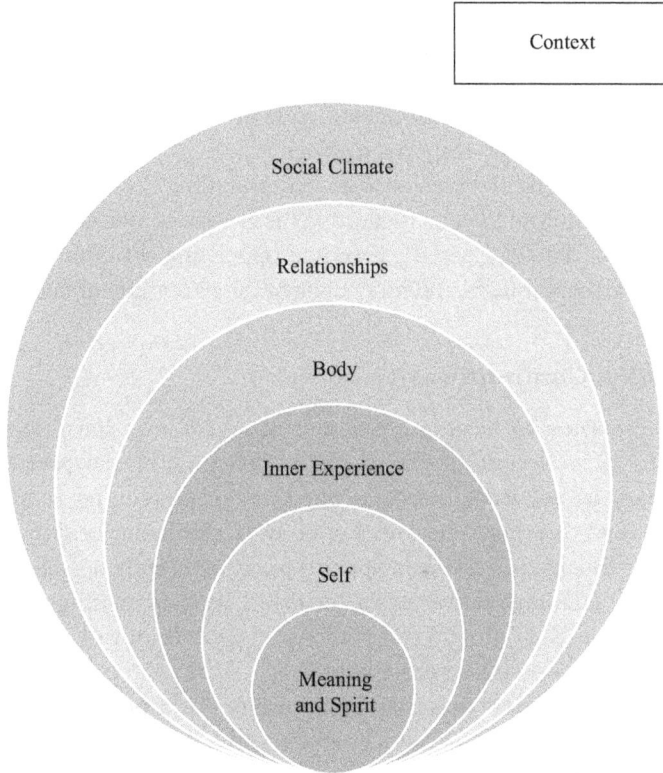

Figure 2.3 Sense of safety: whole person domains.

be threatened by uncertainty, vulnerability, hopelessness and – as we shall see later with Tolstoy's Vronsky – by shame. Our sense of self, our belief in ourselves as worthy of dignity and trust, may be threatened by the suffering we experience,

> whether the vitiating impact of socioeconomic deprivation, the fragmenting effects of sustained domestic violence, the catastrophic consequences of serious disease – or simply the effect of an imbalance between everyday demands and [our] resources to manage.[52]

Our ability to generate and sustain personal meaning and fulfilment, and any spiritual or existential beliefs we may have, can be threatened by any or all of the above, but perhaps particularly by our experiences of grief and loss: this too is an important dimension of Frances' lived experience, and will emerge as a prominent theme in the following chapters on Tolstoy and Hopkins.

And in turn, existential unease can threaten our subsequent physical integrity, as shown in a Norwegian cohort study involving over 20,000 people where unease in the realms of self-esteem, well-being, sense of coherence and social relationships was associated with the subsequent development of multimorbidity in a dose–response manner.[53]

While it is not explicitly oriented to an understanding of suicidal ideation, it is reasonable to infer from Lynch's model that the greater our sense of threat in one or more of these domains, and the fewer our opportunities to find rest, comfort and safety, the more fraught and immediate becomes our dilemma of existence.

Suicide as a Communicative Act

It is also important to recognise that acts of suicide may have implications and significance beyond the individual. Bringing in perspectives from anthropology allows us to consider 'questions of power, the geopolitics of knowledge, and divergent ontologies of body, personhood, health/wellbeing and death'.[54] Suicide may be seen not only as an inherently personal decision but also as a communicative act, a means of sending messages to others; as both an expression of personal choice and as indicator of pathologies of power and larger structural constellations.

These communicative acts may be accusatory at a personal level, as we shall see most vividly in Vronsky's reaction to the death of Anna Karenina. They may be overtly political, as in the tactical employment of suicide bombing by Palestinian combatants, the hunger strikes of Bobby Sands and his fellow republicans in the Maze Prison in Northern Ireland in 1981, or the self-immolation of Jan Palach in Czechoslovakia in January 1969, in protest at the recent Soviet invasion which quashed the democratic energies of the Prague Spring.[55] There may also be no clear boundaries between the personal and the political, as in the cases of indebted Indian farmers whose suicides were widely recognised as symptoms of an ecological, economic and moral crisis in the neoliberal restructuring of Indian agriculture,[56] or of older women from Kerala whose lives are discombobulated by changing domestic economies of care.[57] And, as we will find in Chapter 5, James Joyce and other contemporary novelists show us how even 'everyday suicides' create opportunities for social and moral action and commentary.

Informing Literary Reading

My hope is that, by now, I have offered sufficient access to a set of ideas and tools with which to begin to think critically about how suicidal ideas and actions are portrayed in literary texts. Using Durkheim, Marx and Freud as building blocks, I have indicated the value of a range of sociological, psychological and anthropological perspectives, and suggested how these will impact on my literary analyses in the subsequent chapters.

I am personally drawn to the concept of 'thwarted belongingness' because it seems to me to provide an elegant bridge linking scientific and literary approaches to suicide, exemplifying my intentions in writing this book. Thwarted belongingness captures the essence of the suicidal experience as understood in sociological and psychological theory; at the same time this particular phrasing has rich literary, poetic and novelistic resonance. 'Burdensomeness, defeat, entrapment and strain': all are words which effortlessly bridge the gap between medicine and the humanities, providing points of connection, opportunities for conversation between disciplines which, all too often, find it difficult to know how to approach each other.

We will see how defeat, humiliation and entrapment, and the loss of any sense of safety, lead to tunnel vision and the sense of impending disaster that pervades Anna Karenina's last hours as she heads for the railway station in St Petersburg. And how, over in Dublin, Gerard Manley Hopkins's sense of belonging is hugely thwarted, with deep feelings of loss and separation from family and friends, in hostile, threatening environment very different from home; when these experiences are coupled with intense self-loathing and the perception of burdensomeness, the prospect of ending it all becomes achingly attractive; yet his capability to consider suicide finds expression not in terms of lethal actions but rather through expressions of resolve and endurance.

In the following chapters, I will also show how our encounters with literary texts can illuminate our understanding of suicide beyond even the most well-developed theoretical framework, enabling us to acknowledge the deeply unconsolable and engage with the inadmissible, and thereby building that sense of compassion (and self-compassion) which enables those in the depths of despair to find reasons to stay alive.

Notes

1 Emile Durkheim, *Suicide: A Study in Sociology*, trans. John Spaulding and George Simpson, (London: Routledge, 2005), 243.
2 Ibid.
3 Ibid., 10.
4 Robert Scott, *Scott's Last Expedition: The Journals of Captain R.F. Scott* (London: Pan Books, 2003), 462.
5 Daniel Wilson, 'Evolutionary Epidemiology: Darwinian Theory in the Service of Medicine and Psychiatry'. *Acta Biotheoretica*, 41 (1993): 205–18.

6 Maggie O'Farrell, *Hamnet* (London: Tinder Press, 2020).

7 Jie Zhang, 'Marriage and Suicide Amongst Chinese Rural Young Women'. *Social Forces* 89 (2010):311–26.

8 Karl Marx, *The Economic and Philosophic Manuscripts of 1844*, trans. Martin Milligan (New York: International Publishers, 1964), 182.

9 Bertell Ollman, *Alienation. Marx's Conception of Man in Capitalist Society* (Cambridge: Cambridge University Press, 1971).

10 Karl Marx, ibid., 116.

11 Sigmund Freud, *The Psychopathology of Everyday Life*, trans, Alan Tyson (London: Pelican Books, 1975), 235–36.

12 Sigmund Freud, 'Mourning and Melancholia', in: ed. James Strachey, *The Standard Edition of the Complete Psychological Works of Sigmund Freud* (London: Hogarth Press, 1963) XIV:248.

13 Sigmund Freud. 'Civilization and its Discontents', in James Strachey, ibid. XXI:111, 122.

14 Roland Smith. *Death Drive: Freudian Hauntings in Literature and Art* (Edinburgh: Edinburgh University Press, 2010), 8.

15 Seth Abrutyn and Anna Mueller, 'When Too Much Integration and Regulation Hurt: Re-Envisioning Durkheim's Altruistic Suicide'. *Society and Mental Health* 6, no. 1, (2016):56–71.

16 Anna Mueller et al., 'The Social Roots of Suicide: Theorizing How the External Social World Matters to Suicide and Suicide Prevention'. *Frontiers in Psychology* 12 (2021):621569.

17 Mensah Adinkrah, 'Better Dead Than Dishonored: Masculinity and Male Suicidal Behavior in Contemporary Ghana'. *Social Science and Medicine* 74, no. 4 (2012): 474–81.

18 Robert Merton, 'Social Structure and Anomie'. *American Sociological Review* 3, no. 5 (1938): 672–82.

19 Jie Zhang, 'The strain theory of suicide'. *Journal of Pacific Rim Psychology* 13 (2019):e27

20 Jie Zhang et al., 'Characteristics of young rural Chinese suicides: a psychological autopsy study'. *Psychological Medicine* 40, no. 4, (2010):581–89.

21 Jie Zhang et al., 'When Aspiration Fails: A Study of Its Effect on Mental Disorder and Suicide Risk'. *Journal of Affective Disorders* 151, no. 1 (2013):243–47.

22 Jie Zhang et al., 'Psychological Strains and Youth Suicide in Rural China'. *Social Science and Medicine* 72, no. 12, (2011):2003–10.

23 Bob Lew et al., 'Testing the Strain Theory of Suicide – The Moderating Role of Social Support'. *Crisis* 41, no. 2 (2020):82–88.

24 Thomas Joiner. *Why People Die By Suicide* (Cambridge, MA, US: Harvard University Press; 2005).

25 Derived from Kimberley Van Orden et al., 'The Interpersonal Theory of Suicide'. *Psychological Review* 117, no. 2 (2010):575–600.

26 Antonio Filiberti et al., 'Characteristics of Terminal Cancer Patients Who Committed Suicide during a Home Palliative Care Program'. *Journal of Pain and Symptom Management* 22, no. 1 (2001):544–53.

27 Man-Long Chung et al., 'Predictors of Suicidal Ideation in Social Anxiety Disorder –Evidence for the Validity of the Interpersonal Theory of Suicide'. *Journal of Affective Disorders* 298, Part A (2021): 400–407.

28 Van Orden et al., 'The Interpersonal Theory of Suicide', ibid.

29 Brandon Nichter et al., 'Differentiating U.S. Military Veterans Who Think About Suicide From Those Who Attempt Suicide: A Population-Based Study'. *General Hospital Psychiatry* 72 (2021):117–23.

30 Amy Bohnert et al., 'The Role of Organized Activities in Facilitating Social Adaptation Across the Transition to College'. *Journal of Adolescent Research* 22, no. 2 (2007):189–208.

31 Heather McClelland et al., 'Loneliness As a Predictor of Suicidal Ideation and Behaviour: A Systematic Review and Meta-Analysis of Prospective Studies'. *Journal of Affective Disorders* 274 (2020):880–96.

32 Carol Chu et al., 'The Interpersonal Theory of Suicide: A Systematic Review and Meta-Analysis of a Decade of Cross-National Research'. *Psychological Bulletin* 143, no. 12 (2017):1313–45.

33 Rory O'Connor, 'Towards an Integrated Motivational–Volitional Model of Suicidal Behaviour',in Rory O'Connor et al. eds. *International handbook of suicide prevention: research, policy and practice* (Chichester, UK: Wiley, 2001), 181–98.

34 Based on Rory O'Connor and Olivia Kirtley, 'The Integrated Motivational–Volitional Model of Suicidal Behaviour'. *Philosophical. Transactions of the Royal Society of London B Biological Sciences* 373, no. 1754 (2018): 20170268.

35 Paul Gilbert and Steven Allan, 'The Role of Defeat and Entrapment (Arrested Flight) in Depression: An Exploration of an Evolutionary View'. *Psychological Medicine* 28, no. 3 (1998):585–98.

36 O'Connor and Kirtley, 'Towards an Integrated Motivational-Volitional Model', ibid.

37 Karen Weatherall et al., 'From Ideation To Action: Differentiating between Those Who Think About Suicide and Those Who Attempt Suicide in a National Study of Young Adults'. *Journal of Affective Disorder* 241 (2018):475–83.

38 Thomas Niederkrotenthaler et al., 'Association between Suicide Reporting in the Media and Suicide: Systematic Review and Meta-Analysis'. *British Medical Journal* 368 (2020):m575.

39 Jan Domaradzki, 'The Werther Effect, the Papageno Effect or No Effect? A Literature Review'. *International Journal of Environmental Research and Public Health* 18, no. 5 (2021): 2396.

40 Rory O'Connor et al., 'Psychological Processes and Repeat Suicidal Behavior: A Four-Year Prospective Study'. *Journal of Consulting Clinical Psychology* 81, no. 6 (2013):1137–43.

41 Rebecca Owen et al., 'Defeat and Entrapment in Bipolar Disorder: Exploring the Relationship with Suicidal Ideation from a Psychological Theoretical Perspective'. *Suicide and Life Threatening Behavior* 48, no. 1 (2018):116–28.

42 Karen Wetherall et al., 'An Examination of Social Comparison and Suicide Ideation through the Lens of the Integrated Motivational-Volitional Model of Suicidal Behavior'. *Suicide and Life Threatening Behavior* 49, no. 1 (2019):167–82.

43 Karen Wetherall et al., 'Predicting Suicidal Ideation in a Nationally Representative Sample of Young Adults: A 12-Month Prospective Study'. *Psychological Medicine*, epub ahead of print (2021): 1–8.

44 Derek De Beurs et al., 'Exploring the Psychology of Suicidal Ideation: A Theory Driven Network Analysis'. *Behaviour Research and Therapy* 120 (2019):103419.

45 Johanna Lynch, *A Whole Person Approach to Wellbeing: Building a Sense of Safety* (Abingdon: Routledge, 2021), 94–110.

46 Derived from Lynch, *Whole Person Approach*, ibid., 96.

47 Naomi Godden et al., 'Climate Change, activism, and Supporting the Mental Health of Children and Young People: Perspectives from Western Australia'. *Journal of Paediatrics and Child Health* 57, no. 11 (2021):1759–64.

48 Eugene Tartakovsky and Sophie Walsh, 'Factors Affecting the Psychological Well-Being of Immigrants: The Role of Group Self-Appraisal, Social Contacts, and Perceived Ethnic Density'. *Cultural Diversity and Ethnic Minority Psychology* 26, no. 4, (2020):592–603.

49 Bart Bonikowski, 'Ethno-Nationalist Populism and the Mobilization of Collective Resentment'. *British Journal of Sociology* 68 (2017):S181–213.

50 Erin Toolis and Phillip Hammack, ' "This is My Community": Reproducing and Resisting Boundaries of Exclusion in Contested Public Spaces'. *American Journal of Community Psychology* 56, nos. 3–4 (2015):368–82.

51 Lennox RA. ' "There's Girls Who Can Fight, and There's Girls Who Are Innocent": Gendered Safekeeping as Virtue Maintenance Work'. *Violence Against Women*, epub ahead of print (2021):107780122199878.

52 Christopher Dowrick et al., 'Recovering the Self: A Manifesto for Primary Care'. *British Journal of General Practice* 66, no. 652 (2016):582–83.

53 Margret Tomasdottir et al., 'Does "Existential Unease" Predict Adult Multimorbidity? Analytical Cohort Study on Embodiment Based on the Norwegian HUNT Population'. *BMJ Open* 6, no. 11 (2016):e012602.

54 Daniel Münster and Ludek Broz, 'The Anthropology of Suicide', in Ludek Broz and Daniel Münster, eds, *Suicide and Agency* (London: Routledge, 2020), 8.

55 Karin Andriolo, 'The Twice-Killed: Imagining Protest Suicide'. *American Anthropologist* 108, no. 1 (2006):100–113.

56 Daniel Münster, ' "Farmers" Suicide and the Moral Economy of Agriculture', in Broz and Münster eds, *Suicide and Agency*, ibid., 105–25.

57 Jocelyn Chua, 'Accumulating Death: Women's Moral Agency and Domestic Economies of Care in South India'.in Broz and Münster eds, *Suicide and Agency*, ibid., 147–64.

Chapter 3

ESCAPE FROM THEM ALL
AND FROM MYSELF

She wanted to fall half-way between the wheels of the front truck, which was drawing level with her, but the little red handbag which she began to take off her arm delayed her, and then it was too late. The middle had passed her. She was obliged to wait for the next truck. A feeling seized her like that she had experienced when preparing to enter the water in bathing, and she crossed herself. The familiar gesture of making the sign of the cross called up a whole series of girlish and childhood memories, and suddenly the darkness, that obscured everything for her, broke, and life showed itself to her for an instant with all its bright past joys. But she did not take her eyes off the wheels of the approaching second truck, and at the very moment when the midway point between the two wheels drew level, she threw away her red bag, and drawing her head down between her shoulders, threw herself forward on her hands under the truck, and with a light movement as if preparing to rise again, immediately dropped to her knees. And at the same moment she was horror-struck by what she was doing. 'Where am I? What am I doing? Why?' She wished to rise, to throw herself back, but something huge and relentless struck her on the head and dragged her down. 'God, forgive me everything!' she said, feeling the impossibility of struggling.... A little peasant muttering something was working at the rails. The candle, by the light of which she had been reading that book filled with anxieties, deceptions, grief and evil, flared up with a brighter light, lit up for her all that had before been dark, crackled, began to flicker, and went out for ever.[1]

If you have already read Anna Karenina, this is probably the passage that lodged most powerfully in your memory. And even if you have not yet had the pleasure of Tolstoy's masterpiece, you may well have witnessed this unforgettable scene on film or television, whether performed by Helen McCrory,

Keira Knightley, Sophie Marceau, Nicola Pagett, Tatiana Samoilova or Vivien Leigh, or – first, and for me by far the best – the 1935 interpretation by the incomparable Greta Garbo.[2]

While undoubtedly the most dramatic encounter with suicide in the novel, this is far from the only one. All four of the main characters – Kitty, Vronsky and Levin, as well as Anna – are faced with the question of whether or not they wish to stay alive. I will explore the circumstances that lead each of them to this dilemma, and the different ways in which they respond, bringing to bear not only Tolstoy's own perspectives on suicide (most relevant when considering his near alter-ego Levin) but also the literary and psycho-social insights gained in Chapters 1 and 2. And I will return to Charlie, with whom this book started, whose tragic story has many resonances with Anna's.

Like many other nineteenth-century European authors, including Charles Dickens, Tolstoy first produced the novel in serial form. Thirteen instalments were published in the periodical *Russian Messenger* between January 1875 and April 1877. It was very well received at the time and there was considerable frustration amongst the reading public when the last instalment, covering the story after Anna's death, was delayed for several months while Tolstoy and the journal editor resolved a major disagreement over his expression of anti-nationalist views.

I can neither read nor translate Russian, so have been content to rely on the work of others in accessing Tolstoy's writings. Amongst the many excellent English translations of Anna Karenina in existence, I have noted those by Rosemary Edmonds 1954 version (my own first introduction to the text), Rosamund Bartlett's more recent offering from 2014, and the 2003 translation by Richard Pevear and Larissa Volokhonsky, which is widely respected for its attention to precise literal accuracy. I have chosen to refer primarily to the 1912 translation by Louise and Aylmer Maude, who benefited from direct correspondence with Tolstoy himself and whose text provides a highly readable, narrative flow. On occasions I discuss alternative translations, and draw on further advice from my academic colleague Josie Billington.

It's All So Unimportant

Kitty, formally Princess Ekaterína Alexándrovna, is the third daughter of Prince Alexander Scherbástky. She is 18 and in her first season in Moscow high society. Expected to make a match with a man of her social standing, she falls in love with Count Alexei Vronsky, an army cavalry officer who has been paying her a great deal of attention. When aristocratic landowner Konstantin Levin, her long-term suitor, arrives at her home to ask for her hand in marriage, she turns him down, believing that Vronsky is about to propose to her. At the big society ball she attends later that same day, Kitty is on tenterhooks, waiting on an imminent declaration of love from Vronsky. She is shocked and heartbroken when she realizes that he has fallen for Anna instead, and that his apparent interest in her was nothing more than a passing, inconsequential flirtation.

> Kitty was for a moment seized with despair. She had refused five men who had asked for the mazurka [so that Vronsky could invite her] and now she had no partner for it [...] She must tell her mother she was feeling ill, and go home, but she had not the strength to do it. She felt herself quite broken-hearted.[3]

Kitty goes into a grave, potentially terminal decline for several months, and can see no way out. In a darkly comedic example of the medicalization of human misery,[4] Tolstoy describes how doctors are consulted, a tubercular condition is suspected as the cause of her failing strength, nervous excitation and lack of appetite. Cod-liver oil and iron supplements are prescribed, and her mother proposes a trip abroad in remedy. Kitty knows this is all absurd.

> Her whole illness and the treatment seemed to her stupid and even ridiculous. Her treatment seemed to her as absurd as piecing together the bits of a smashed vase. Her heart was broken. Why did they want to dose her with pills and powders?[5]

Eventually, Kitty and her mother decide to travel to a small German spa, or watering place. Kitty forms a close friendship with Varenka, the adopted daughter of the pietistic Madame Stahl. While she finds temporary relief from her own suffering in following Varenka's example in caring for other sick people at the spa, the main benefit for Kitty is the opportunity she has to share her distress about her failed love affair. Varenka's tale of her own reciprocated love for a man whose mother forced him to marry someone more suitable encourages Kitty to express directly how insulted, angry and ashamed she was by Vronsky's rejection.

> 'But the humiliation?' said Kitty. 'One cannot forget the humiliation, one cannot', and she remembered the look she gave Vronsky at the ball, when the music stopped.
> 'Where is the humiliation? You did not do anything wrong?'
> 'Worse than wrong, shameful.'
> Varenka shook her head and put her hand on Kitty's.

'Shameful in what respect?' she said. 'You could not have told a man who
was himself indifferent to you that you loved him?'

'Of course not; I never said a single word, but he knew it. No, no; there
are such things as looks and ways of behaving. If I live to be a
hundred I shall never forget it.'

'Why does it matter? I don't understand. The question is, do you love him
now or not?' said Varenka, calling everything by its plain name.

'I hate him; I cannot forgive myself.'

'But what does it matter?'

'The shame, the humiliation.'

'Dear me, if every one were as sensitive as you are!' said Varenka.
'There is no girl who has not gone through the same sort of thing.
And it is all so unimportant.'[6]

This conversation (illustrated on the cover of this book by the artist Zahar
Pichugin) provides Aristotelian catharsis for Kitty. It is the first time that
she has been able to talk openly and share her genuine, heartfelt emotions
with another sympathetic human being. In ways prescient of the tenets of
cognitive-behavioural therapy, Varenka listens attentively, takes Kitty's
concerns seriously, offers her comfort (placing her hand on Kitty's); all
while challenging her negative perceptions and conclusions.[7] Twice she asks
So what then?, pushing Kitty to articulate precisely what her grievances are.
And the final *it's all so unimportant*, which could be interpreted as belittling
or trivializing her trauma, in the context of the conversation and their
relationship as a whole has a radically different effect, enabling Kitty to see
that there could conceivably be a world of worth and value beyond Vronsky
and that no-longer fateful evening at the ball.

Varenka's help gives Kitty the courage finally to see that she is not Varenka,
and cannot be her (as she had wished to be): she can only live by her own
heart. Despite never finding out what Varenka does consider to be important,
and despite some turbulence in their relationship, Kitty remains close
friends with Varenka. They agree to meet again if and when she marries.
She returns home to Russia. 'She was not as carefree and light-hearted
as before, but she was at peace. Her old Moscow sorrows were no more than
a memory'.[8] Her existential crisis is over.

So as Not to Be Ashamed

Count Alexéi Kiríllovich Vronsky – known familiarly as Alóysha – has two
encounters with suicide over the course of the novel. The first is in his sitting
room in St. Petersburg. He has returned home after visiting his lover Anna

who, having safely given birth to their daughter, has developed a severe puerperal fever and is on the verge of death. But this is not the only, or indeed the principal cause of his distress. Speaking in her delirium, believing that she is dying, Anna has begged her husband Alexei Alexandrovich Karenin to forgive not only her but also Vronsky:

> 'Remember that the only thing I want is your forgiveness, I wish for nothing else…. Why does he not come in?' she cried, calling to Vronsky on the other side of the door. 'Come, come! Give him your hand.'
> Vronsky came to her bedside and, seeing Anna, again covered his face in his hands.
> 'Uncover your face! Look at him! He is a saint', said she. 'Uncover, yes, uncover your face!' she went on angrily. 'Alexei Alexandrovich, uncover his face! I want to see him.'
> Karenin took Vronsky's hands and moved them away from his face, terrible with is look of suffering and shame.
> 'Give him your hand. Forgive him […].'
> Karenin held out his hand, without restraining the tears that were falling.
> Thank God, thank God', she cried, 'now everything is ready.'

Karenin escorts Vronsky off the premises: 'If she wishes to see you I will let you know; but now I think it will best better for you leave'.

On the porch of the Karenin's house, and later in his own sitting room, Vronsky reflects on the multiple sources of his deep unhappiness. He realizes he loves Anna more than ever before, yet has now lost her forever. He understands Karenin to be magnanimous and himself in the wrong: he has been humiliated before her, 'leaving her nothing but a shameful memory of himself'. Worst of all was 'the ridiculous, shameful figure he had cut when Karenin was pulling his hands from before his shame-suffused face'.

He can no longer see any value in his life. Things he thought he held dear – his army career, his position in high society – no longer matter. His mind goes around in circles, from lost happiness, to the meaningless of his life, to his sense of humiliation.

> 'This is how one goes mad' he said again, 'and how one shoots oneself so as not to be ashamed.'[9]

He takes his revolver from his table, turns it to a loaded chamber, and shoots himself in the chest.

To his intense embarrassment, Vronsky misses his heart. He survives, with the help of his brother's wife Varya. While convalescing he claims he shot himself accidentally and insists Varya tells everyone the same, 'Or else it would be too stupid'. But to himself, the shooting is now as an act of cleansing, of contrition. He has washed himself of his humiliation and once again has 'found he could look people in the face once more, and [....] live in accord with his former habits'.[10] He decides to get away from St. Petersburg and applies for a military posting in Tashkent.

Here, we have a fascinating series of reflections on Vronsky's motives for this impulsive (though very serious) attempt to kill himself. He believes he has lost his lover, not once but twice: first because she is going to die, and second because she has renounced him for her husband. His main response to this is not overwhelming grief but rather a sense of humiliation: her last memory of him will be a disgraceful one, while in her eyes her husband is now elevated to the level of a saint. But what he finds worst is the realisation that Karenin has not only regained Anna's love but also – and most insupportable – attained a relational, social and moral victory over him. To take an analogy with primate behaviour in evolutionary biology,[11] in this battle between two alpha-males Vronsky has lost, and lost badly. The image of Karenin taking his hand in forgiveness, and exposing his distress and weakness in the process, is too much for him to bear. He has been firmly (if very politely) banished. Shame and humiliation are his drivers to suicide. Although Karenin's forgiveness is real, and for him the alpha-male battle may be (albeit temporarily) irrelevant, it remains devastatingly important to Vronsky. They may be inhabiting separate mental universes, but can still damage one another in the same world.

This analysis is confirmed by his reactions during his recovery. There is no mention of any inconsolable sadness at the loss of Anna. The only concerns he expresses to himself are a sense of relief that his actions have absolved him of any sense of humiliation, and that he can now face his peers in society without shame.

In relation to the theories of suicidal behaviour discussed in Chapter 2, while acknowledging some elements of thwarted belongingness, it is evident that Vronsky's suicidal impulses are primarily egotistic in the Durkheimian sense,[12] prompted by losing his stake in his community, and by his sense of humiliation and defeat. And there is a strong resonance with Freud's death instinct, his assertion that 'men are not gentle creatures who want to be loved [...] they are on the contrary, creatures amongst whose instinctual endowments are to be reckoned a powerful share of aggressiveness'.[13] Here, the aggression between himself and Karenin is played out in highly sophisticated ways, leaving the only person that Vronsky can attack to be himself.

This is also a classic illustration of the critical role of shame in the theories of Mueller and Abrutyn.[14] Vronsky's sense of identity is deeply embedded in his position within the elite officer corps of the Imperial Army. He is committed to this identity above all else, and has a significant emotional attachment to the social ties it offers him. So, his failure, which he sees not so much in terms of the apparent ending of his relationship with Anna as in terms of his humiliation at the hands of Karenin, leads him to a profound sense of shame, since he judges himself – and assumes others similarly judge him – to be deficient. As a result, he fears that his essential social connections are in danger of dissolution or loss.

Odd though it may seem, Tolstoy himself expressed surprise at Vronsky's suicide attempt. As a prime example of how authors are not necessarily control of their characters, in a letter to his friend Nicolai Strakhov in April 1876, he wrote:

The chapter about how Vronsky accepted his role after meeting the husband had been written by me a long time ago. I began to correct it, and quite unexpectedly for me, but unmistakably, Vronsky went and shot himself. And now it turns out that this was organically necessary for what comes afterwards.[15]

It is indeed the case that this (to Vronsky) shameful episode provides a fitting antithesis to his second encounter with suicide, which is less direct and considerably less impulsive.

After Anna's death, Vronsky is distraught. He joins a group of Russian volunteers to fight in the Orthodox revolt that has broken out in Serbia against the Turkish Empire. We find him departing by train from St. Petersburg. We first see him through the eyes of Anna's brother 'His face, which was aged and full of suffering, seemed petrified'. Then, we are party to an account from Vronsky's mother: 'For six weeks he spoke to no one and ate only when I implored him to. One could not leave him a moment alone. We took away everything that he could kill himself with.' She believes the war has been sent by God to lift her son up again, but Vronsky's reality is quite the reverse. In conversation with Levin's brother, he reveals that his clear intention in volunteering is to put himself in the Turk's firing line, in the hope of easeful death:

No introductions are needed to enable one to die. [...] As a man I have this quality, that I do not value my life at all and that I have physical energy enough to hack my way into a square and slay or fall – that I am sure of. I am glad that there is something for which I can lay down the life which I not only do not want, but of which I am sick! It will be of use to somebody.

The narration then passes to Vronsky himself. Standing by the side of the railway he has a flashback to the moment when he finds Anna's blood-covered body 'stretched out shamelessly before the eyes of strangers', her face frozen in an expression 'pitiful on the lips and horrible in the fixed open eyes – an expression which repeated, as if in words, the terrible phrase about his repenting it – which she had uttered during their quarrel'.

Try as he might to remember his best moments with her – and there were many – he cannot do so. His life has been for ever poisoned by their last, bitter unresolved argument, and by the knowledge that she has finally triumphed over him, leaving him with futile but 'irrevocable remorse'.[16] The phrasing of this in Pevear and Volokhonsky's more recent translation – 'ineffaceable regret' – is elegant, with 'ineffaceable' bringing to mind the literal impossibility of Vronsky's forgetting Anna's face, and 'regret' mirroring her final words to him. However, I prefer the Maude translation of Tolstoy's original text as 'remorse', which encompasses Vronsky's sense of guilt at the pain he caused Anna during her final days and hours.

One again he has lost love, this time certainly more prominently than before. But once again, also, he has the overwhelming sense of defeat, this time inflicted not by Karenin but directly and deliberately by Anna herself, and as a result all the harder to bear. Although there are several points in the novel where Tolstoy's opening epigram – 'Vengeance is mine; I will repay' – could apply, for me this is the central one. Anna (as we shall soon see) felt betrayed by Vrosnky's behaviours towards her, his apparent coldness and his supposed infidelities. For Vronsky, there is nothing here of the inexplicability of suicide, which was such a prominent theme in Chapter 2. In his mind the reasons for – and consequences of – Anna's death are all too painfully clear: she has taken her revenge in the most powerful and permanent way possible. He no longer has any sense that his life has intrinsic worth; his old world-view has crumbled and he is unable to reconstitute it in ways that give him reason to stay alive. Actively seeking out 'death by soldiering' allows him to retain his sense of honour, his alpha-maleness, performing actions that may conceivably prove of value to others. There is now a degree of Durkheimian altruism at play. With the apparent nobility of his impending self-sacrifice, he is also avoiding any recurrence of that sense of shame that was so devastating to his self-esteem after his earlier failed suicide attempt. It is reminiscent of Kevin Costner charging the Confederate lines in the opening sequences of the film *Dances with Wolves* and – perhaps – with the modern phenomenon of 'suicide by cop'.[17] It is his only way out.

You Will Regret This

Anna Arkádyevna Karenina (formerly Princess Oblonsky) has her first direct encounter with the dilemma of her own existence when she is pregnant with Vronsky's child, while still living with and married to Alexei Karenin. Anna's dearest wish would be to divorce Karenin and marry Vronsky, while continuing to have the care of her beloved son Seroyzha. But she knows this to be impossible. Under Russian law at that time, divorce could only be instigated by the innocent party (in this case Karenin), who would automatically take custody of any children of the marriage. The tensions in this triangular – or rather quadrilateral – relationship are acute and frequently unbearable for her. While not actively contemplating suicide, she sees her impending death in childbirth as an honourable way of resolving her dilemma.

In conversation with Vronsky, she explains what she believes is going to happen.

> 'Soon, very soon, everything will get disentangled and we shall be able to rest and not torment each other any more.'
> 'I do not understand', he said, though he did understand.
> 'You were asking when? Soon, and I shall not survive it. Don't interrupt!' she said hurriedly. 'I shall die, and I am very glad that I shall die: I shall find deliverance and deliver you.'

Anna goes on to recount her vivid – and recurring – dream of 'a peasant with a rough beard, small and dreadful. I wanted to run away, but he stooped over a sack and was fumbling in it [....]'

> 'He fumbles about and mutters French words, so quickly, so quickly, and with a burr, you know: "*Il faut le batter, le fer: le broyer, le pétrir*" (You must beat the iron, pound it, knead it). And in my horror I tried to wake, but I woke still in a dream and began asking myself what it could mean; and Korney [her servant] says to me "You will die in childbed, in childbed, ma'am..." Then I woke.'
> 'What nonsense, what nonsense!' said Vronsky, but he felt that there was no conviction in his voice.[18]

In fact, Vronsky had the same dream himself, just a few days earlier, so is disposed to believe her interpretation of it. And, as we have seen, Anna's prediction nearly comes true, as she develops (but eventually survives) a severe infection after the birth of her daughter.

Given what is to follow for Anna, the option of death at this point might, as Andrei Zorin suggests[19], have been preferable for her. Despite her initial belief that she can make her marriage with Karenin work, she finds that she cannot bear living with him, his forgiveness of her and his attachment to her baby daughter Annie become intolerable. Becoming desperate at the prospect of Vronsky's departure, she reunites with him. They elope to Europe with the prospect of divorce from Karenin, leaving her son Seryozha behind.

From here on her life slowly, but inexorably, crumbles around her, in ways that allow for a multitude of interpretations. Psychologically, she is unable to square the circle between her own 'unpardonable happiness' and her knowledge of her husband's unhappiness. As Josie Billington argues compellingly, her need to dismiss Karenin, her analogy of the 'drowning man who has torn away another man clinging to him' so that the other is drowned, is at one level 'the only salvation'.[20] But this reflex expulsion and denial of painful thoughts about her husband, about the evil she has done to him and about her own sense of guilt, have deeply serious, long-term consequences for her inner being, for her soul.[21]

The recurrent nightmare of the French-speaking peasant continues to haunt her. For Vladimir Nabokov, this peasant symbolizes 'what her sinful life has done to her soul – battering and destroying it – [...] now she will follow the direction of her dream and have a train, a thing of iron, destroy her body'.[22] More sympathetically, Gary Browning proposes the phallic imagery of these nightmares, the iron-beating, to represent the remorseless power of male sexuality; and argues that Anna comes to believe that both of her French-speaking men, Karenin and Vronsky, view her as no more than an inanimate, unfeeling object, subjecting her to relentless emotional and physical abuse.[23]

Socially, she finds herself isolated and ostracized, especially in the grand salons of high metropolitan society, most spectacularly at her ill-fated visit to the theatre in St. Petersburg. This progressively affects her relationship with Vronsky, who can still move freely in social circles, and has his military career and his estate to occupy him. Her boredom, and her dependence on him engender bitterness and cause the couple to argue endlessly. She becomes pathologically jealous, accusing him of multiple affairs. She turns to morphine to help her sleep.

According to both the Interpersonal Theory[24] and the Integrated Motivational-Volitional (IMV) model[25] which I explored in my Chapter 2, Anna fulfils *all* the criteria for high suicidal risk. Her belongingness to her life's loves, whether Vronsky or her son Seryozha, now seems to her to be entirely thwarted. She perceives herself as an insupportable burden to Vronsky, who at the same time is her only possible source of solace and support, both emotional and material. She feels lonely and disconnected, in the absence of any reciprocally-caring relationships. She feels defeated, humiliated and trapped, with no possibility of escape or rescue. She ruminates endlessly on her life's difficulties, and has little belief in the possibility of solving her problems. Following Zhang, we can also see that her values are under severe strain,[26] especially in the unresolvable conflict between her desires for Vronsky and Seryozha. And by now she is constantly under threat; there is nowhere, other perhaps than the opium bottle, where she even momentarily feels safe.[27]

Images of death present themselves to her clearly and vividly

> as the sole means of reviving love for herself in his heart, of punishing him, and of gaining the victory in the contest which an evil spirit in her heart was waging against him. [...] When she poured out her usual dose of opium and thought that she needed only to drink the whole phial in order to die, it seemed to her so easy and simple that she again began thinking with pleasure how he would suffer, repent and love her memory when it was too late.[28]

These thoughts are temporarily displaced by her terror of death and her joyful belief that he does, after all, still love her. They discuss returning from Moscow to their country estate, where they have been happier, but she hesitates, uncertain of his motives. They launch into their final argument. Anna's last words to him 'You [...] you will repent of [regret] this'[29] are seen by Vronsky as an improper, irritating threat. He decided to pay no attention, and leaves to visit his mother.

How many domestic arguments end exactly like this?

There then follow some of the most remarkable pages in modern literature, reminiscent of (though of course pre-dating) both James Joyce and Virginia Woolf, as we witness Anna's last few hours of life through her stream of complicated, contradictory and ultimately self-destructive consciousness. For me this passage is the most compelling and authentic literary example of what Al Alvarez describes as the 'shabby, confused, agonised crisis which is the common reality of suicide'.[30] It is compulsive – and I would suggest compulsory reading – for anyone wishing to understand the experience of another human being in deepest distress. It is the passage that prompted me to write this book.

The Zest Is Gone

Anna panics after Vronsky's departure, sending him first a handwritten note – 'I was to blame. Come home. We must talk it over. For God's sake come; I am frightened!' and then a telegram *I must speak to you, come at once*. In scenes reminiscent of Romeo and Juliet, receipt and response to these messages are confused and misinterpreted. The world is closing in on her. She travels by carriage, first for a frenetic visit to Kitty and her sister Dolly, then to the railway station, with the intention of finding or exposing Vronsky. She wrongly assumes animosity from Dolly and Kitty, food disgusts her, her servants irritate her, 'Everything is nasty'.

On the way to the station she ruminates about Vronsky: 'What did he look for in me? Not so much love as the satisfaction of his vanity'. Everything she sees out of her carriage window confirms the futility of life, not only for herself but for those she passes by. '*The zest is gone!* [...] Every effort has been made, but the screws have given way.... A beggar woman with a baby. She thinks I pity her. Are we not all flung into the world only to hate each other, and therefore to torment ourselves and others?'.

She now even questions the reality of her love for her son 'I thought I loved too, and was touched at my own tenderness for him. Yet I lived without him and exchanged his love for another's'.

Moment to moment, she oscillates between hope and despair. She sees a funny hairdresser's sign and thinks she will share a laugh about it with Vronsky, but then realizes she may never seem him again. At the station everyone looks ugly or stupid. She is irritated by the superficial conversation of a husband and wife. She sees a dirty ugly peasant in a peaked cap bending down to the wheels of a railway carriage and terrifyingly recalls her dream. Vronsky isn't there, and she rejects his 'careless' final note, thinking to herself 'No, I will not let you torture me'. Everyone on the platform seems to be talking about or looking at her, so she moves along to get away from them.

Once again, death seems to be the answer. In phrasing reminiscent of Macbeth's final soliloquy, she asks herself: 'Why not put out the candle, if there's nothing more to look at? If everything is repulsive to look at it? [...] It's all untrue, all lies, all deception, all evil! [...]'

'Suddenly remembering the man who had been run over the day she first met Vronsky, she realized what she had to do'. She walks to the end of the platform, down the stairs to the railway track, stopping close to a passing goods train, and estimates the midpoint between the front and back wheels. 'There, into the very middle, and I shall punish him and escape from everybody and from myself'.[31]

It is important to point out that 'escape from' is only one possible translation of this key phrase, which, as Josie Billington notes, fits well with the sense of punishment for its urgency and resentment. Tolstoy's root verb also translates as 'to be saved from' or 'be rid of' (as in the Pevear and Volokhonsky version), reflecting Anna's desperation to vacate her situation, and perhaps closer to her tragic evasiveness. And from the related noun, Billington also offers the translation of 'deliverance'[32] which, when linked with 'saved', may even allow the inclusion of an oblique religious meaning to her last few words.

And then we are into the final paragraph (presented in full at the beginning of this chapter), with her memory of diving into water, her recollection of past joys, her horror and recoil, her begging for forgiveness, the peasant muttering over his iron, her candle flaring, sputtering and going out.

Throughout the years Tolstoy spent creating his novel, he struggled in his relationship with the character of Anna. Her fate was suggested early on, by a real incident in 1872 when he saw the body of a local woman (also called Anna) who hurled herself under a goods train after her lover abandoned her. In earliest versions of the text he expressed greater sympathy with the saintly Karenin, and portrayed Anna as the type of married woman in society who ruins herself. Suicide was a punishment not only for her adultery but also for what was to Tolstoy, a political and religious radical but highly conservative when it came to gender roles, the unforgivable sin of taking contraceptive measures to remain physically attractive to Vronsky.[33] Yet it is a sign of his genius as a writer, and his extraordinary ability to generate compassion for his characters, that he draws ever closer to her as the story unfolds; so that, in these final moments of her fictional life, it becomes virtually impossible to distinguish between character and novelist.

My principle reflection at this point is a reminder that – as we shall see later with Sylvia Plath – Anna's suicide was not inevitable, but almost casual. Although the world was closing in on her, although everything and everybody seemed vile, it could have been averted. Just because it *did* happen, it does not follow that it *had to* happen. There were choices and contingencies, right up to the last few seconds of her life. She oscillated between despair and hope in her carriage. As John Bayley notes at her amusement over the hairdresser's name

> Quite unexpectedly Tolstoy makes us feel that if anything could have saved Anna it would have been her own sense of comedy and the absurdity of life, and the simple wish to share a joke with her lover.[34]

If Vronsky had received her first message sooner, and responded differently. If the irritating couple had not entered her railway carriage. If the people standing on the platform had not critically commented on her costume, forcing her to walk to the end of the platform. It was only in those last few minutes that 'she realized what she must do'. Like Vronsky's decision to shoot himself, this was an impulsive act.

For me as a clinician, and as a human being, Tolstoy's message here is critical: even in the most desperate of circumstances, even if we are convinced that the whole world is against us, until that very last moment when the train actually rolls over us, the possibility of hope remains.

This thought gives me solace, when I reflect on the life and death of Charlie, whom I introduced at the very beginning of this book. You may recall that she used to be the singer in a band, but for many years had suffered from chronically low self-esteem, continually reinforced by long-term abuse from her ex-partner; that she had recently been diagnosed with breast cancer secondaries in her spine; that her consequent anxiety and depression, self-treated but also exacerbated by alcohol, led her to take several overdoses; and that her attempts to start a new life for herself, with the support of many good friends, were frustrated by forced isolation during the first major lockdown of the COVID-19 pandemic.

The fear and loneliness became too much for her. She took another overdose, survived it, but kept on drinking. She reached out to her son in the hope of a few seconds conversation with her beloved granddaughter Tammy, but her call was blocked.

Two days later she was dead.

Liver damage, from a combination of secondary cancer and alcohol, caused the blood vessel in her oesophagus to rupture, leading to catastrophic internal bleeding. The police were called and found her in bed, lying in a congealed pool of blood. On her table was an opened copy of Michael Moorcock's *The Sundered Worlds*. Beside her on the bed were two photographs: one of her young self, singing with the band; the other of her and Tammy, all dressed up at a family celebration, smiling joyously together. These potent images were the last she ever saw: her life as it had been; her life as she wished it to be; but her life that was to be no more.

Like Anna, Charlie was at very high risk of suicide. Her belongingness to her life's loves, especially her granddaughter Tammy, now seemed to her to be entirely thwarted. She felt lonely and disconnected, in the absence of any reciprocally-caring relationships. She felt defeated, humiliated and trapped, with no possibility of escape or rescue. Her chronically low self-confidence meant she too easily assumed herself to be a burden to the many people who reached to offer her care and support, and left her with little belief in the possibility of solving her problems. And her previous overdoses had demonstrated her capability of suicide, her ability to tolerate the related fear and pain. She had the strain of being unable to find the coping skills to address the crises engulfing her. And in addition, her sense of safety[35] was overwhelmed by the multiple threats to her existence; there was nowhere, other perhaps than the vodka bottle, where she even momentarily felt safe.

Although technically, legalistically, this was not suicide but accidental death, for me and for Charlie such differences are semantic and irrelevant. She could no longer find any reasons to stay alive. Her hope was extinguished.

We might assume, as with Anna, that her tragic end was inevitable, that the constellation of adverse circumstances meant Charlie's death, was one way or another, imminent. It is indeed true that the advanced nature of her cancer meant her life would be foreshortened. Yet the timing – and the manner – of her passing could so easily have been different. If the pandemic had not forced her into complete isolation, away from the therapeutic comfort of her friends. If her son had not refused her contact – even a few minutes on Zoom – with her beloved granddaughter. She might have found the grace to stay alive, to keep her flame of hope alight.

He Acted and Lived Unfalteringly and Definitely

Konstantín Dmítrich Levin – known familiarly as Kóstya – faces none of the dilemmas of existence that confront and eventually overwhelm Anna. His roles in life, as a man, as an aristocratic landowner, as husband to Kitty and father of many children, are socially accepted and unimpeded. He experiences no sense of shame in his social relations. He is able to love his wife, his family and his children without compromise, secrecy or ambiguity. He is confronted with no impossible choices about whom he should spend his time with. He experiences no stigma, no external pressures to behave differently and no humiliation. His belongingness is not thwarted. He does not perceive himself to be a burden to those around him. He is neither trapped nor defeated.

Yet we find him, in the final chapters of the novel, in the depths of despair.

> And although he was a happy and healthy family man, Levin was several times so near to suicide that he hid a cord he had lest he should hang himself, and he feared to carry a gun lest he should shoot himself.[36]

It is more or less impossible to distinguish here between Levin and Tolstoy himself, since the author endows the character with his own biographical details and personality traits. During the 1850s, and even more so during the 1870s while writing *Anna Karenina*, Tolstoy experienced prolonged periods of melancholic distress. My introduction to Leo in Chapter 1 could equally be an introduction to Levin, while passages of Tolstoy's *Confession*[37] could equally be transposed verbatim into the final chapters of the novel. So, I will make no apologies for conflating the two in my discussion of the cause and resolution of the dilemma of his existence.

The explicit trigger, the precipitating factor, for Levin's despair – the sight of his beloved brother Nikolai dying – mirrored Tolstoy's own distress at the death of his elder brother (also Nikolai) from tuberculosis, and would surely have reactivated his longstanding grief at the loss of his mother in his early childhood. In addition, during the period when he was writing the novel, Tolstoy had to face the death of a favourite niece, three of his own children (the oldest only 17 months) and two of the aunts who had cared for him during his childhood. It may well be, as I suggested in Chapter 2, that Freud's mechanisms of mourning and melancholia[38] are at work here, with grief, loss and anger turning inwards on himself. We also read that Levin's distress was perpetuated and deepened after his wife gave birth, 'while he was living idly in Moscow', a reminder that, for Tolstoy, sophisticated metropolitan society was an unwanted interference in the realities of rural life; and perhaps evidence of a sense of strain between two differential value systems.[39]

The form that this dilemma takes for Levin, as for Tolstoy, is of profound existential uncertainty, a threat to his sense of safety because of his inability to generate personal meaning and fulfilment, or any sustaining spiritual beliefs.[40] He is horrified not so much at death 'than by life without the least knowledge of whence it came, what it is for, why, and what it was'. His attempts to replace his childhood religious faith with modern ideas of science and philosophy, feel like 'a person who has exchanged a thick fur coat for muslin garment and who, being out in the frost for the first time, becomes clearly convinced, not by arguments, but with the whole of his being, that he is as good as naked and that he must inevitably perish miserably'.

Pinning his hopes on materialist philosophies feels like 'seeking for food in a toyshop or at a gunsmith's'. Moral philosophers such as Plato, Spinoza and Schopenhauer offer him some temporary understanding and relief, as do the writings of the Slavophile religious philosopher and poet Khomiakov, but then 'suddenly the whole artificial edifice tumbled down like a house of cards'.[41]

At this point Levin's subjective experiences, albeit derived from radically different causes, begin to mirror those of Anna. He feels the cruel mockery of some evil and offensive power. He is 'in painful discord with himself'. 'Without knowing what I am and why I'm here, it's impossible for me to live. And I cannot know that, therefore I cannot live.' He had 'either to explain his life so that it did not look like the wicked mockery of some devil, or shoot himself'. In such moments both Anna and Levin are deeply conflicted, with no sense of the safety or reality of their being in the world, and hence utterly alone. As Richard Pevear observes, 'Metaphysical solitude is the hidden connection between them, and is what connects them both to the author'.[42]

But, unlike Anna, 'he did not hang or shoot himself and went on living'.[43] Why?

There seem to me to be two separate, though interrelated dimensions to Levin's (at times highly precarious) ability to avoid killing himself and to carry on living. In consideration of the fundamental question behind this book, which is whether literary reading can help people considering suicide to stay alive, I would suggest that both are important, either may be sufficient, but only the first is strictly necessary.

The first way in which Levin (and Tolstoy) is able to stay alive is by doing rather than thinking.

> When Levin thought about what he was and why he lived, he could find no answer and was driven to despair; but when he left off asking himself these questions, he seemed to know what he was and why lived, for he acted and lived unfalteringly and definitely.[44]

For me the crucial phase here is 'when he left off asking himself these questions'. His endless ruminations, however erudite they may be, are getting him nowhere except to dig himself deeper and deeper into the well of his despair. Instead, just focusing on the business of everyday life is what gets him through: '[...] it seemed to him that he had to do what he was doing'. He finds he is able to work through his suicidal impulses by active, wholehearted engagement in his customary pursuits. Returning to his country estate from Moscow, he becomes involved in and occupied by managing his estates, by the hard physical activity of cultivating his own land himself, cutting deeper and deeper into the soil, like a plough, by his passion for beekeeping, by his conversations with peasants, neighbours and visiting relatives, by his daily interactions with his household and family, by his concerns about Kitty and baby being in danger from a storm-damaged oak tree, and by the need for him to arrange a washstand in the bedroom of his newborn son Sergei.

It is worth noting that this approach to managing distress, this focus on activity rather than cognition, is the basis of the therapeutic intervention known as behavioural activation: an approach that aims to increase engagement in adaptive activities, especially those associated with the experience of pleasure or achievement, and to solve problems in a rewarding way.[45]

Just as Kitty and Varenka engage in a de facto CBT session while at the spa in Germany, Levin is here creating a behavioural activation programme for himself, through this series of practical and social activities – of which beekeeping is likely the most valuable to him – that bring him enjoyment or a sense of accomplishment. There is good evidence that such an approach is an effective treatment for depression.[46] And his energetic physical exercise, in the form of agricultural labour, not only brings him metaphysical benefit in terms of his desire to connect with the land and with the 'genuine life' of the local peasants, but may also have a direct physiological impact in reducing his emotional distress.[47]

I will extend this line of inquiry further in Chapter 6, when considering whether our engagement in the ordinary activity of our everyday lives, our commitment to the circumstances in which we find ourselves, may be crucial to the existential preservation of the self.

Serving the Universe

The second dimension to Levin/Tolstoy's survival is an emergent spiritual understanding. This begins with his realization that reasoning is of no help to him at all, but that if he stops thinking, and simply lives, he finds a moral purpose or judgement to guide his actions:

> But when he did not think, but just lived, he unceasingly felt in his soul the presence of an infallible judge deciding which of two possible actions was the better and which the worse; and as soon as he did what he should not have done, he immediately felt this.[48]

Knowledge of what is good cannot be explained by reason, he decides; goodness sits outside the chain of cause and effect. He understands that 'his life was good, but his thinking was bad'. Then his conversation with Theodore, a religious peasant, about a morally upright old man who lives for the soul and remembers God, has, like Paul on the road to Damascus, 'produced in his soul the effect of an electric spark'. The point of his existence is to serve the good, to 'live not for one's needs, but for God!'[49]

Daily life intrudes for a while. Levin finds himself irritated with the driver of his gig, and involved in pointless arguments with his brother and a visiting philosopher. But despite all that,

> returning into that mood, he felt with joy that something new and important had occurred within him. Reality had temporarily veiled the spiritual tranquility he had found, but it remained with him.
>
> Just as the bees, now circling around him, threatening him and distracting his attention, deprived him of complete physical calm and forced him to shrink to avoid them, so the cares that had beset him from the moment he got into the trap had deprived him of spiritual freedom; but that continued only so long as they surrounded him. And as, in spite of the bees, his physical powers remained intact, so his newly-realized spiritual powers were intact also.[50]

For Tolstoy, as here for Levin, life is never simple. At first, he thinks he just has to re-embrace his old religious beliefs, but he soon realizes that will not quite work for him. His revelation of living not for one's own needs but for God is immediately, in the next sentence followed by the three-word question 'For what God?'

It is at this point that Levin and Tolstoy begin to separate. In the final pages of the novel, Levin sees the main proof of God being his 'revelation of what is good', which 'can always be verified in my soul'. His whole life now 'is no longer meaningless as it was before, but has an unquestionable meaning goodness with which I have the power to invest it'.[51] But before he can formulate the answer to what exactly his revelation may be, or explain the unquestionable meaning of the good, he finds himself busy in the nursery with Kitty, discussing washstands and attending to the needs of baby Sergei.

In one sense, for present purposes, this is an entirely sufficient resolution. Tolstoy is telling us that seeking to do good in the world is what gives us meaning, overcomes our despair, addresses our dilemma of existence and gives us reason to stay alive. But moving beyond the text of *Anna Karenina* and into his subsequent and overtly religious writings, we find what Tolstoy has in mind, which is no less than a radical rewriting of Christianity.

In a letter to his friend Nikolai Strakhov, written in November 1877, he writes that he would like to be a *yurodivy* – 'God's fool'[52] – a wandering beggar, often of low intelligence, who embodies ideals of poverty and asceticism historically observed in Christianity, and in many other religious traditions. His many attempts to live like this involved himself in endless disagreements with his wife Sofia, as he repeatedly renounced his substantial worldly privileges and goods.

Over the next few years, he develops, as Andrei Zorin puts it 'a comprehensive religious, moral, political, social and economic philosophy that was stunning it its logic and consistency'.[53] In his 1884 essay *What I Believe*, he proposes that the doctrine of Christ consists of five commandments: never condemn anyone or regard anyone as an outlaw; do not commit adultery, including divorce and remarriage; do not swear oaths, pledge loyalty to earthly governments or participate in legal proceedings; do not resist evil with violence and do not regard other human beings as enemies or aliens.[54]

Amongst this complex combination of beliefs, ranging from social conservatism in marriage to radical anti-state anarchism and the abolition of the division of mankind into nations, what stand out for me are his commitments to social justice and to non-violence. Using his position as the most famous living novelist in the world, he collected more than a million roubles in international donations, principally from Quakers in the United States and Britain, and set up hundreds of field kitchens to feed many thousands of the people affected by the terrible famine of 1891. His belief in non-violence – expressed most cogently in his later book *The Kingdom of God Is Within You*[55] – inspired many around the world, not least Gandhi, who corresponded with him in 1909 and 1910[56] while advocating for Indian rights in the South African Transvaal, and generated his related concept of *satyagraha*, a force born of truth and love of non-violence.

As well as doing much good in the world, this outworking of Tolstoy's revised Christian doctrine was of benefit to him personally. Although he continued – perpetually – to question and doubt himself, he never again experienced the intensity of anguish, the existential despair, that left him with a hold on life scarcely less precarious than Anna's or Levin's.

Suicide becomes not just a problem of the past for Tolstoy, but a morally indefensible action. Writing to a friend in 1898, he addresses the question 'Has a man in general the right to kill himself?' He acknowledges that the possibility of killing oneself is a safety-valve, and that man continually uses this right when he kills himself in duels, in war (like Vronsky), or by tobacco, wine (in part like Charlie) or opium (in part like Anna). But he now argues that it is neither reasonable nor moral to do so. Life is beyond time and space; death will 'arrest its manifestation in world' but we do not know (like Hamlet's 'dread of something after death') whether its manifestation in another world will be more or less pleasant. We deprive ourselves of the experiences that could be acquired in this world. And we have no right to assume that the object of our life is our own pleasure, rather than to offer service to others.

He tells the story of a paralysed monk who lived joyfully for 30 years, giving inspiration to many thousands, and commands his friend that

> Life in its entirety, and the possibility of living until natural death, have been given to man only on the condition that he serve the life of the Universe. But, having profited by life so long as it was pleasant, he refuses to serve the Universe as soon as life becomes unpleasant: whereas, in all probability, his service commenced precisely when life began to appear unpleasant. All work appears at first unpleasant. [....] While there is life in man, he can perfect himself and serve the Universe. But he can serve the Universe only by perfecting himself, and perfect himself only by serving the Universe.[57]

Although these appear to be his final written words on the question of suicide, I am not for a moment wishing to present this letter of Tolstoy's as the definitive answer. Indeed, I feel decidedly uncomfortable with it, and would prefer that he had not written it. But there it is: he did. As you may have gathered by now, I feel more at home in the realms of existential uncertainty which he inhabits with his characters in *Anna Karenina*. Tolstoy's tone in this letter is highly reminiscent of Stevie Smith, who we will see in Chapter 5 chiding her audience and herself to 'prate not of suicide', and to 'study to deserve death'. It may be that, like Smith, he is protesting too much, arguing against some residual doubts inside himself. Or it may be that his position here is simply the logical extension of his now firmly held beliefs in the existence of a providential God within a caring universe. In either event, I profoundly disagree that perfection is or should be our aim; it is an impossibility, and seeking it only serves to reinforce a sense of failure. Instead, let us join Samuel Beckett in failing again, and failing better.

My concluding reflections on this chapter are fivefold. First and probably most important is that, in *Anna Karenina*, Tolstoy has gifted us some of the most evocative, compelling and empathic descriptions of suicidal thoughts and actions ever written, providing deeply compassionate insights not only for those who live with such experiences but also for those who care for them. Second is the invaluable reminder that suicidal action is not an inevitable consequence of suicidal ideas, even in the most extreme circumstances. Third is the suggestion that our contemporary theories of suicidal ideation may not adequately account for the extent of potential motivating factors, such as Vronsky's shame and humiliation or Levin's existential despair. Fourth is the realization that there are effective ways of resolving our dilemmas of existence available to us without necessary recourse to health professionals, whether it be through the cognitive-behavioural approach taken by Varenka for Kitty, or Levin's self-created versions of behavioural activation and exercise therapy. And finally, there is Tolstoy's proposal to look beyond the self and seek to do good in the world. Whether this needs to derive from a belief in the divine, and if so should take the form of radical Christian anarchism, remain moot points. But in either event, it sets us up well for our next exploration, into the theologically charged poetry of Gerard Manley Hopkins.

Notes

1 Leo Tolstoy, *Anna Karenina*, trans. Louise and Aylmer Maude (London: Everyman's Library 1912, 1992), 904–905.
2 Anna Karenina's death scene as portrayed on film. Accessed 25 February 2021. https://www.youtube.com/watch?v=G-uRIOFrmO4.
3 Tolstoy, *Anna Karenina*, ibid., 96.
4 Christopher Dowrick and Allen Frances, 'Medicalising Unhappiness: New Classification of Depression Risks More Patients Being Put on Drug Treatment from Which They Will Not Benefit'. *British Medical Journal* 347 (2013):f7140.
5 Tolstoy, *Anna Karenina*, ibid., 141.
6 Tolstoy, *Anna Karenina*, ibid., 262–63.
7 Brian Sheldon, *Cognitive-Behavioural Therapy: Research, Practice and Philosophy*, (London: Routledge, 1995).

8 Tolstoy, *Anna Karenina*, ibid., 279.

9 Tolstoy, *Anna Karenina*, ibid., 488–93.

10 Tolstoy, *Anna Karenina*, ibid., 511.

11 Patrik Lindenfors and Birgitta Tullberg, 'Evolutionary Aspects of Aggression the Importance of Sexual Selection.' *Advances in Genetics* 75 (2011):7–22.

12 Emile Durkheim, *Suicide: A Study in Sociology*, trans. John Spaulding and George Simpson (London: Routledge, 2005), 243.

13 Sigmund Freud, 'Civilization and its Discontents', in: ed. James Strachey, *The Standard Edition of the Complete Psychological Works of Sigmund Freud* (London: Hogarth Press, 1963), XXI, 111.

14 Anna Mueller et al., 'The Social Roots of Suicide: Theorizing How the External Social World Matters to Suicide and Suicide Prevention.' *Frontiers in Psychology* 12 (2021):621569.

15 Leo Tolstoy, 'Letter to N N Strakhov, 23 and 26 April 1876', in *Tolstoy's Letters: Volume 1 1828–1879*, selected, edited and translated by Reginald Christian (London: Athlone Press, 1978), 297.

16 Tolstoy, *Anna Karenina*, ibid., 913–20.

17 Kris Mohandie et al., 'Suicide by Cop Among Officer-Involved Shooting Cases.' *Journal of Forensic Sciences* 54, no. 2 (2009):456–62.

18 Tolstoy, *Anna Karenina*, ibid., 427–28.

19 Andrei Zorin, *Leo Tolstoy* (London: Reaktion Books, 2020), 96.

20 Tolstoy, *Anna Karenina*, ibid., 463–64.

21 Josie Billington, *Is Literature Healthy?* (Oxford: Oxford University Press, 2016), 21–23.

22 Vladimir Nabokov, *Lectures on Russian Literature* (New York: Harcourt Brace Jovanovich, 1980), 175

23 Gary Browning, 'Peasant Dreams in Anna Karenina'. *The Slavic and East European Journal* 44, (2000), 525–36.

24 Kimberley Van Orden et al., 'The Interpersonal Theory of Suicide.' *Psychological Review* 117, no. 2 (2010):575–600.

25 Rory O'Connor. 'Towards an Integrated Motivational–Volitional Model of Suicidal Behaviour'. In Rory O'Connor et al. eds. *International Handbook of Suicide Prevention: Research, Policy and Practice* (Chichester, UK: Wiley, 2001), 181–98.

26 Jie Zhang. 'The Strain Theory of Suicide'. *Journal of Pacific Rim Psychology* 13 (2019):e27

27 Johanna Lynch, *A Whole Person Approach to Wellbeing: Building a Sense of Safety* (Abingdon: Routledge, 2021).

28 Tolstoy, *Anna Karenina*, ibid., 884.

29 Tolstoy, *Anna Karenina*, ibid., 886.

30 Al Alvarez, *The Savage God: A Study of Suicide* (Bantam Edition: Random House New York. 1973).

31 Tolstoy, *Anna Karenina*, ibid., 888–904.

32 Josie Billington, Personal communication, 7 March 2021.

33 Zorin, *Tolstoy*, ibid., 96: with reference to Leo Tolstoy, *Anna Karenina*, ibid., 637–39.

34 John Bayley, 'Preface', in: Leo Tolstoy L, *Anna Karenina*, ibid., ix.

35 Lynch, *Whole Person Approach*, ibid.

36 Tolstoy, *Anna Karenina*, ibid., 930.

37 Leo Tolstoy, *A Confession and Other Religious Writings*, trans. Jane Kentish (London, Penguin Book, 1987).

38 Sigmund Freud, 'Mourning and Melancholia', in *Standard Edition*, ibid., XIV:248.

39 Jie Zhang, 'Strain Theory of Suicide', ibid.

40 Lynch, *Whole Person Approach*, ibid.

41 Tolstoy, *Anna Karenina*, ibid., 926–28.

42 Richard Pevear, 'Introduction', in: Leo Tolstoy, *Anna Karenina*, trans. Richard Pevear and Larissa Volokhonsky (Penguin Books: London 2000), xx.

43 Tolstoy, *Anna Karenina*, ibid., 930.

44 Tolstoy, *Anna Karenina*, ibid., 789–90.

45 Sona Dimidjian et al., 'The Origins and Current Status of Behavioral Activation Treatments for Depression'. *Annual Review of Clinical Psychology* 7, no.1 (2011):1–38.

46 Pim Cuijpers et al., 'Behavioral Activation Treatments of Depression: A Meta-Analysis'. *Clinical Psychology Review* 27, no. 3 (2007): 318–26.

47 Mandy Hu et al., 'Exercise Interventions for the Prevention of Depression: A Systematic Review of Meta-Analyses'. *BMC Public Health* 20, no.1 (2020):1255.

48 Tolstoy, *Anna Karenina*, ibid., 993.

49 Tolstoy, *Anna Karenina*, ibid., 936–937.

50 Tolstoy, *Anna Karenina*, ibid., 804.

51 Tolstoy, *Anna Karenina*, ibid, 959,963.

52 Tolstoy, *Letters Volume 1*, ibid., 308.

53 Zorin, *Tolstoy*, ibid., 113.

54 Leo Tolstoy, *What I Believe*, trans. Constantine Popoff, (New York: Gottsberger, 1886), accessed 18 March 2021. https://archive.org/details/WhatIBelieve_109/mode/2up.

55 Leo Tolstoy, *The Kingdom of God Is Within You*, trans. Aline Delano (London: Walter Scott, 1894).

56 Leo Tolstoy, 'Letters to Mohandas Gandhi, 8 October 1909 and 7 September 1910', in *Tolstoy's Letters: Volume II 1880–1910*, selected, edited and translated by Reginald Christian (London: Athlone Press, 1978), 692, 706–08.

57 Leo Tolstoy, *Letter on Suicide*, accessed 22 February 2021. https://en.wikisource.org/wiki/Tolstoy_letter_on_Suicide.

Chapter 4

NOT CHOOSE NOT TO BE

I first met Gerard Manley Hopkins when I was 18, living in a hostel in West Bromwich. I was there as a community service volunteer for eight months between leaving school and starting university. I had recently split up with my girlfriend. I knew nobody at all in the area. I was desperately lonely. One evening I stood for a while, looking over the edge of a motorway bridge, wondering what it would be like to jump off.

Someone – I wish I could remember who – gave me a copy of Robert Bridge's selection of Hopkins' poetry,[1] and there I found poem 41:

> No worst, there is none. Pitched past pitch of grief,
> More pangs will, schooled at forepangs, wilder ring.
> Comforter, where, where is your comforting?
> Mary, mother of us, where is your relief?
> My cries heave, herds-long; huddle in a main, a chief-
> Woe, wórld-sorrow; on an áge old anvil wince and sing -
> Then lull, then leave off. Fury has shrieked 'No ling-
> ering! Let me be fell: force I must be brief'.
>
> O the mind, mind has mountains; cliffs of fall
> Frightful, sheer, no-man-fathomed. Hold them cheap
> May who ne'er hung there. Nor does long our small
> Durance deal with that steep or deep. Here! creep,
> Wretch, under a comfort serves in a whirlwind: all
> Life death does end and each day dies with sleep.

These one hundred and twenty-six words resonated so strongly with me, not for any hope they offered (though as we shall see, there may be a little hidden in here), but because I'd found somebody else who felt like I did, had been there himself, was talking my language, who had experienced and shared my anguish and distress, my sense of devastating emptiness. Alongside frequent late-night listenings to the final *adagio lamentoso* from Tchaikovsky's

Symphonie Pathétique,[2] with its fading into nothingness, Hopkins' poem somehow kept me going. I owe him a lifelong debt of gratitude.

He has been my frequent companion, sometimes haunting but more often inspiring me, ever since. He regularly finds his way into my writings and lectures, including my contribution to Josie Billington's *Reading and Mental Health*[3]; and my related series of blogposts on 'sonnet therapy' in which I propose a course of six of his sonnets as guides on a journey from despair to delight.[4]

In this chapter, I will take the opportunity to extend these thoughts, through a more detailed analysis of the turmoil Hopkins expresses in his so-called terrible sonnets, and consider what they can tell us about the dilemma of existence, about staying alive despite suicidal despair.

But first, some background on Hopkins' life and poetic vision.

Simple and Beautiful Oneness

Hopkins was born in Stratford, Essex in 1844, the eldest of probably nine children. His father worked in marine insurance, wrote poetry and was at one stage consul-general for Hawaii. Gerard was brought up in a strong Anglican tradition, and as a boy was accomplished at drawing, violin and mathematics. He read Classics at Balliol College Oxford between 1863 and 1867, where he began his lifelong friendship with Robert Bridges, and had a brief but intense emotional engagement with Bridges' younger cousin Digby Dolben, who died by drowning two years later. In 1866, he converted to Roman Catholicism, a radical step at the time and one which led to long-term disagreements with his family and many of his former friends.

Within the Catholic church he decided to become a Jesuit. Following training in London, Stonyhurst in Lancashire and St. Beuno's in north Wales, he was eventually ordained as a priest in 1877. For a while he gave up writing poetry, believing it to be antithetical to his religious vocation. He changed his mind while at Stonyhurst, after being introduced to the medieval theologian Duns Scotus, whose concept of the 'univocity of being', that words used to describe the properties of God may equally be used to describe people or things, enabled him to realise that his poetry and spiritualty were complementary.

Hopkins was fascinated by the structure of poetics, especially of the sonnet, like the Italian poet and scholar Francesco Petrarca (Petrarch) and William Shakespeare before him. Like Petrarch (but unlike Shakespeare) he usually divided his sonnets into two parts: the first eight lines or octet setting out the main theme, with the last six lines offering a response. Sometimes the octet is divided thematically into two sets of four lines, or quatrains. His octets have a rhyming structure *abba abba*, with the sestets rhyming variably, for example *cdc dcd* or *ccd ccd*. Like both Petrarch and Shakespeare, Hopkins' standard format is the iambic pentameter, 10 syllables in a line, with the stress placed on each second syllable: 'I <u>wake</u> and <u>feel</u> the <u>fell</u> of <u>dark</u>, not day'. Each set (for instance, 'I wake') is a foot or iamb. However, he enjoyed experimenting with the length and rhythm of his lines.

He invented the concept of sprung rhythm, with feet composed of between one and four syllables, with the intention of reflecting the dynamic quality of normal speech and natural phenomena. Usually he kept the standard five stressed syllables per line, but the number of unstressed syllables (and therefore line length) can vary, as in the first two lines of 'The Windhover':

> I <u>caught</u> this <u>mor</u>ning <u>mor</u>ning's <u>min</u>ion <u>king-</u>
> dom of <u>day</u>light's <u>dau</u>phin, dapple-<u>dawn</u>-drawn <u>Fal</u>con, in his <u>rid</u>ing

Sometimes he included an extra foot, which he calls an <u>outride</u>: as in [<u>Felix</u> <u>Ran</u>dal] [the <u>far</u>rier], [O is he] [<u>dead</u> then]? [my <u>duty</u>] [all <u>end</u>ed].

And in three poems – one of which was 'Ash Boughs', which he wrote during the same period as his 'terrible sonnets' – he brings his early love of mathematics into play by inventing an entirely new form, the curtal sonnet, whose ten-and-a-half lines are structured proportionately as three-quarters of a full sonnet.

In his journals he coined the term *inscape*. Inscape is the charged essence, the absolute singularity that gives each created thing its being, the unified complex of characteristics that give each thing its uniqueness and that differentiate it from other things. His complementary term *instress* refers both to the energy that holds the inscape together and – importantly – the impulse from the inscape which carries it whole into the mind of the beholder.[5]

> There is one notable dead tree [...] the inscape markedly holding its most simple and beautiful oneness up from the ground through a graceful swerve below (I think) the spring of the branches up to the tops of the timber. I saw the inscape freshly, as if my mind were still growing, though with a companion the eye and the ear are for the most part shut and instress cannot come.[6]

Building on the theology of Duns Scotus, for Hopkins inscape and instress describe the overflowing presence of the divine within the temporal. The unique thingness of a thing equates to its sanctity, its purpose in the world. Hopkins presents this most perfectly in 'The Windhover', composed just a few months before his ordination, with his vision of the dapple-dawn-drawn falcon riding effortlessly through the air. I shall return to this wonderful poem later in the chapter.

His clerical duties took him to several parishes across Britain, including a period in Liverpool between December 1879 and August 1881. St. Francis Xavier in Salisbury Street was at that time the largest and one of the poorest Catholic parishes in England, and (another point of personal connection for me) is just a few minutes' walk from my University office. He found life here very tough, writing to a friend – in terms reminiscent of Frederick Engels' descriptions of Salford in the 1840s – of

> a truly crushing conviction of the misery of town life to the poor and more than to the poor, of the misery of the poor in general, of the degradation even of our race, of the hollowness of this century's civilisation.[7]

He was able to create a few poems while he lived here, most notably 'Felix Randal', in tribute to one of his parishioners, a blacksmith, 'big-boned and hardy-handsome', who died of pulmonary tuberculosis at the age of 31 (the average life expectancy in Liverpool at that time[8]). This poem resonates strongly with me as a modern general practitioner, not only with its vivid descriptions of Felix's physical decay, 'Pining, pining, till time when reason rambled in it, and some/Fatal four disorders, fleshed there, all contended', but also in recognition of the mutual benefits for Hopkins and his parishioner that derived from his care of Felix as his death approached. 'This seeing the sick endears them to us, *us too it endears*'[9] [my emphasis]: the acknowledgement that we ourselves receive comfort as we offer comfort to others.

In February 1884, Hopkins moved to Dublin to take up the appointment of Professor of Greek and Latin at University College, a position he held until his death from typhoid fever on 8 June 1889. It was during this period, most likely between late 1884 and September 1885, that he wrote the six sonnets which are the focus of this chapter.

A Continually Jaded and Harassed Mind

Hopkins finds life difficult in Dublin, which by the time he arrives has faded from its former Georgian elegance. He is not enjoying his work, comprising in large part of marking examination scripts, and is concerned about the effects of fail marks on the future careers of his students. His physical health is suffering. He feels a long way from home, both culturally and geographically. He is worried by the level of political agitation and anti-English sentiment in the city, including a 'monster meeting' at nearby Phoenix Park in March 1885. And around this time, he learns of the deaths of two former friends from his Oxford undergraduate days, Tom Nash and Martin Deldart, both assumed likely to be suicides.

All these problems take their toll. On 17 May 1885, he writes to his barrister friend Alexander Baillie, reporting that 'this melancholy I have all my life been subject to has become more of late years not indeed more intense in its fits but rather more distributed, constant and crippling'.[10] And in a letter to Robert Bridges, written on the same day, he apologises for his recent silence due to

work, worry and languishment of body and mind – which must be and will be; and indeed to diagnose my own case (for every man by forty is his own physician or a fool) [...] well then to judge of my case, I think that my fits of sadness, though they do not affect my judgement, resemble madness.

He goes on to report 'I have after long silence written two sonnets, which I am touching: if ever anything was written in blood one of these was.'[11] This sonnet 'written in blood' may have been 'Carrion Comfort', or else 'I Wake and Feel'[12].

By beginning of September his mood is a little lighter, having spent some time in England, visiting family and friends. He writes to Bridges 'I have just returned from an absurd adventure which, when I resigned myself to it I could not help enjoying'. The assumption that he is referring to his mental adventures is supported later in the letter when he writes

I shall shortly have some sonnets to send you, five or more. Four[13] of these came like inspiration, unbidden and against my will. And in the life I lead now, which is one of a continually jaded and harassed mind, if in any leisure I try to do anything I make no way – nor with my work, alas! But so it must be.

He is convinced he is producing nothing of poetic value, and that he is destined 'to be time's eunuch and never to beget'. His holiday has given him 'some buoyancy' but he fears he will soon 'be ground down to a state like this last spring's and summer's, when my spirits were so crushed that madness seemed to be making approaches'.[14]

None of these six sonnets were published in Hopkins' lifetime. Bridges waited almost thirty years after his death, until 1918, before including them in the first major edition of his poetic works. The phrase 'terrible sonnets' was never used by Hopkins himself. Bridges referred to them as 'terrible posthumous sonnets', while Gardner described them as 'sonnets of desolation'. There has been a lively debate about the precise timing or order in which he wrote them, and whether they can be assumed to form a narrative arc.[15] Daniel Harris and Hillis Miller argue vigorously that they cannot, and should be read collectively as evidence of 'a hideous despair [...] an experience of chaos scarcely duplicated elsewhere',[16] or a 'shattering experience of the disappearance of God'.[17] However, I am inclined to side with Norman White[18] and Paul Mariani[19] that they can justifiably be read as offering insights not only into his experience of despair and suicidality but also his routes through and out of it; providing not just a narrative arc but also a therapeutic trajectory.

Bearing in mind the evidence from his letters that his 'languishment of mind' of the spring was replaced by a certain 'buoyancy' by early autumn of 1885, and acknowledging that there can be no certainty of Hopkins' intentions, I choose to explore these six sonnets in the following order: 'To Seem the Stranger', 'No Worst, There is None', 'I Wake and Feel', 'Carrion Comfort', 'Patience' and 'My Own Heart'. Several commentators have suggested that this order closely follow the classical descent and ascent of the spiritual exercises of Ignatius Loyola, founder of the Jesuits, and hence may indicate deliberate correspondence on Hopkins' part.[20,21,22] This interesting proposition is beyond the scope of my present enquiries.

My Lament Is Cries Countless

The first three sonnets in this set – 'To Seem the Stranger', 'No Worst, There is None' and 'I Wake and Feel' – collectively cover the range of theories of suicidal ideas and behaviours that I introduced in Chapter 2. Like Tolstoy's descriptions of Anna's last hours, and Levin's existential crisis, they provide us with profoundly disturbing yet astonishingly lucid insights into the world of a person in extreme despair.

In 'To Seem the Stranger', Hopkins works through four degrees of separation, which he calls 'removes'.

The first is from his family, in consequence of his conversion to Catholicism.

> To seem the stranger lies my lot, my life
> Among strangèrs. Father and mother dear,
> Brothers and sisters are in Christ not near.

The second is from his country, where the predominantly Protestant population remains deeply suspicious of Catholic doctrine.

> England, whose honour O all my heart woos, wife
> To my creating thought, would neither hear
> Me, were I pleading, plead nor do I: I wear-
> y of idle a being but by where wars are rife.
> I am in Ireland now; now Í am at a third
> Remove.

His third remove is geographical and political, across the sea to Ireland at a time of highly charged debate over independence, 'where wars are rife'. His fourth and final degree of separation, his most telling alienation, is not social but spiritual:

> Only what word
> Wisest my heart breeds dark heaven's baffling ban
> Bars or hell's spell thwarts. This to hoard unheard,
> Heard unheeded, leaves me a lonely began.[23]

He wants to offer his wise words to the world but, despite everything he has done for his God, he is barred by 'dark heaven's baffling ban', or perhaps thwarted by 'hell's spell'.

Within Durkheim's typology of suicides, Hopkins in Dublin fits the egotistic type, with little social integration, a sense of not belonging, of having no stake in the community.[24] We also see a Marxian sense of alienation, as a sensuous, suffering, passionate being with a profound sense of social dislocation.[25] Following Mueller and Abrutyn, his 'identity renders painful the possibility of exclusion, rejection, and isolation from cherished social groups'.[26] And with Zhang, he is experiencing strain from differential values, between his beliefs and those of his family and his country, and from the discrepancy between his aspirations and (what he perceives as) the reality of his situation.[27] In 'disillusioned recognition of powerlessness'[28] he realises that his hoard of knowledge and wisdom is unheard; even if it is heard, then it remains unheeded and ignored, not only by his family and others but also by God himself. At the end of this sonnet, Hopkins finds himself back at the beginning, and at a point where, despite all his remarkable linguistic talents, he becomes almost inarticulate with exasperation.[29]

In 'I Wake and Feel' he cries for help, but there is none to be found.

> And my lament
> Is cries countless, cried like dead letters sent
> To dearest him that lives alas! away.

The 'dearest him' might be his good friend and regular correspondent Robert Bridges, but is more likely to be Jesus, with the dead letters his unanswered prayers; his phrasing resonant with the Book of Lamentations, 'Also when I cry and shout, he shutteth out my prayer',[30] and with the psalmist's complaint that 'You have taken from me friend and neighbour/darkness is my closest friend'.[31]

'Comforter, where, where is your comforting?' he asks in 'No Worst', 'Mary, mother of us, where is your relief?' His 'cries heave', but there is no answer. His belongingness is utterly thwarted; he is a burden to others, causing strife within his family.[32] His sense of social, relational and spiritual safety are all under threat.[33] He is absolutely alone.

This may all seem intolerable enough, but there is more to come.

'No Worst, There is None' offers a series of graphic external, physical and geographical metaphors, prefaced by the horrific realisation that like Edgar in King Lear, he cannot say 'This is the worst.' There is no worst. Like the overpowering waves of a stormy sea or the unrelenting gusts of a hurricane, his pangs of grief come back at him, time and time again. He is huddled like a herd of cattle, caught in the eye of a storm. He is battered on an anvil (very different from the creative one used by blacksmith Felix Randal in Liverpool) and at the mercy of evil furies. He is in full awareness of his 'wórld-sorrow'; the same pain that in German is called *Weltschmerz* and is close to the Buddhist noble truth of *dukkha*: the sadness of simply existing in a world of suffering and transience.

We follow him upwards into the mountains of his mind, and then over his 'cliffs of fall/Frightful, sheer, no-man-fathomed', on his downwards spiral into chaos. He is losing 'grasp of his own modes of sensory perception'.[34] By now he is trapped and entirely defeated.[35] He warns us 'Hold them cheap/ May who ne'er hung there'. Indeed: his 'descent into the dizzying depths of the self'[36] is anything but cheap, as anyone who has experienced even a glimpse of the dislocating power of grief can testify.

And we are provided with yet further images of distress, when Hopkins wakes and feels 'the fell of dark, not day'. 'Fell' here has multiple meanings, all of them highly relevant. It is the past tense of 'fall', which in theological terms denotes a sense of original sin; it can mean something deadly, of terrible evil or ferocity; it can mean the coarse skin, hide or pelt of an animal, so the physical sense of being smothered; and he may also be using it in the sense of a now-obsolete word to signify gall, anger and bitterness.

His gaze is now is on the infinite slowness of time. The light is permanently delayed. Never-ending darkness stretches out for hour upon hour upon hour, into all his Macbethean tomorrows, across the years to the last syllable of recorded time.

> What hours, O what black hoürs we have spent
> This night! what sights you, heart, saw; the ways you went!
> And more must, in yet longer light's delay.
>   With witness I speak this! But where I say
> Hours I mean years, mean life.

Unlike Jean Paul Sartre, who finds a sense of shelter in being alone with his sorrow, where his solitude creates 'a bleak wall, a little darkness to screen us from that bleak immensity' of the 'absolute monotony of the world',[37] there are no redeeming features in Hopkins' darkness. For him it is an impermeable separation from the light he still believes in, even though he can no longer gain access to it.

In the sestet of 'I Wake and Feel', linking back to one of the meanings of 'fell', Hopkins moves on to physical – or more precisely gastro-intestinal – experiences of suffering:

> I am gall, I am heartburn. God's most deep decree
> Bitter would have me taste: my taste was me;
> Bones built in me, flesh filled, blood brimmed the curse.
> Selfyeast of spirit a dull dough sours. I see
> The lost are like this, and their scourge to be
> As I am mine, their sweating selves; but worse.[38]

In Sartre's novel, *Nausea*, his central character Antoine Roquentin, like Hopkins living with the intense desolation of being entirely alone, also experiences this overwhelming physical sensation of nausea. Roquentin finds his nausea existentially reassuring, as proof that he exists:

> There is bubbling water in my throat, it caresses me - and now it comes up again into my mouth. For ever I shall have a little pool of whitish water in my mouth – lying low – grazing my tongue. And this pool is still me. And the tongue. And the throat is me.[39]

But there is no such consolation for Hopkins. His nausea and heartburn are 'God's most deep decree/ Bitter would have me taste: my taste was me'. He remains a son of Adam, 'whose blood brimmed the curse' in the Garden of Eden. And 'Selfyeast of spirit a dull dough sours'. He is no more than the bitter taste in his own mouth, souring his food with his own dulled spirit.

It Brings a Closeness

By now we could be forgiven for assuming that these sonnets are, in effect, a series of suicide notes, and that Hopkins is beyond all hope of recovery. But this is not entirely the case. Even in these bleakest of his sonnets, moments of hope, of other possibilities, can be found. The classic structure of the sonnet, with the octave setting out the theme and the sestet providing a response, provides the opportunity for a degree of balance between despair and optimism.

In 'To seem the Stranger', he acknowledges that 'in all removes I can/ Kind love both give and get'. He may be religiously estranged from his family, but they are still on cordial terms. As with his time in Liverpool, he can find mutual support with those he meets in Dublin. The final lines of 'No Worst' offer some (admittedly scant) comfort, first in the injunction 'Here! creep/ Wretch under a comfort serves in a whirlwind'. This may be an allusion to God calling to Job out of a storm, demanding to know why he is obscuring his plans with words without knowledge,[40] a suggestion that there may after all be some purpose behind all this horror. And he has the thought that these terrible experiences cannot last forever, since 'all/ Life death does end and each day dies with sleep'. Perhaps there is some equivalence here with the temporary relief to be had from the 'rough comforter [or quilt] he can pull over his head there in his bleak upper-story room on dank St. Stephen's Green'.[41] And in 'I Wake and Feel', Hopkins offers two more elements of relief. Although he may be alone, he is finding some inner company. Within the first three lines, he switches from the first person 'I' to 'we' (I plus heart) and then to 'you' (heart). He is not dealing with all this on his own. His heart is taking some of the burden for him. And in the final lines of this sonnet we have 'I see/The lost are like this, and their scourge to be/ As I am mine, their sweating selves; *but worse* [my emphasis]'. As with God in the whirlwind, there may be some reason for his suffering: to gain an empathic insight into the eternal torment of those in hell, which is worse than his own because he has not yet lost all hope of recovery.

This is one way in which these sonnets, terrible though they may be, can offer help to someone wondering whether or not to stay alive, or to someone else wishing to support someone in that frame of mind. Even in the depths of despair, there remains the possibility of something different: that we can still find moments to give and receive kindness; that it cannot be never-ending;

or that there may perhaps be some purpose behind it all. We do not have to share Hopkins' views on the afterlife to gain value from this last idea. If we have experienced grief and loss ourselves, we are so much better placed to offer empathy and compassion to those going through it now.

There are other tangible benefits to be found here. They offer us a connection, as my 18-year old self found when I first discovered 'No Worst' in my room in thehostel. There was a link for me, a sense of shared experience with Hopkins.

Frances is the lonely civil servant, whom I introduced in Chapter 1. She lives by herself with her cat, Danny. She finds the business of getting through life immensely difficult, and sees her existence as a never-ending, bleak monotony. She is a good friend to others but doesn't like to share her problems with them. I know she is a regular attender at her local Catholic church, and finds comfort in her faith, so it occurs to me that she may be sympathetic to Hopkins' work.

During one of our regular consultations, I tentatively suggest that she has a look at some of these sonnets. When she comes for her next appointment with me, she brings her own copy of his selected poems with her. 'It's like finding a friend', she tells me; 'I felt like he was sitting next to me, reading to me. It brings a closeness.' Paradoxically, witnessing his aloneness enables her to feel less alone.

These sonnets also help us to realise that it is legitimate to feel so distressed, something we may often doubt or even feel guilty about. Reflecting on her reactions to 'No Worst' and 'I Wake and Feel', Frances tells me she has spent far too much time berating herself for feeling as unhappy as she does, when there seems to be no good reason for it. Her present life is ostensibly fine, she has a good, full-time, rewarding job, her companion cat Danny, is involved with her local Catholic church, and has friends she can visit whenever she chooses. But now she can see that it is permissible for her past experiences of trauma to still have an effect on her emotions:

It's allowed, you're entitled to feel that depth.

There is something powerful, impressive and inspirational about Hopkins' absolute, raw honesty here, his ability to give deep expression to the reality of his experiences, however terrifying that reality may be. There is no pretence, no denial and no hiding. As Brett Beasley comments,

His ability to use form as a way of channelling and bearing witness to angst while refusing to explain it away or let it evaporate into abstract knowledge was as unparalleled in his time as it is in our own.[42]

At the same time, there is an element of detachment. Despite his obvious distress, Hopkins is able to write perfectly formed classic sonnet lines: 5 feet, 10 syllables, with the stress on every second one: 'I <u>wake</u> and <u>feel</u> the <u>fell</u> of <u>dark</u> not <u>day</u>'. In the sestets he can choose to vary his rhyming structure from *cdc dcd* in 'To Seem the Stranger' (third/can/word; ban/unheard/began) and *No Worst* (fall/cheap/small; creep/all/sleep), switching to *ccd ccd* (decree/me/curse; see/be/worse) in 'I Wake and Feel'. And it is worth remembering that he also composed 'Ash Boughs', his mathematically arranged curtal sonnet (exactly three-quarters of the length of a standard sonnet) during this period.

For the past few years, I have been practising mindfulness meditation on a regular basis. And this is precisely the point where mindfulness begins, resting in the present moment, however difficult that moment happens to be, paying attention to our thoughts and feelings and to the world around us. Mindfulness teaches us to observe our thoughts and feelings as temporary events, rather than reflections of the self that are necessarily and permanently true. We learn to stay with and acknowledge the present reality of our situation, without judgment or evaluation. Without avoiding any of the problems we face, or trying to solve them: just being there.[43] We begin to find an at first infinitesimal but gradually expanding sense of detachment, a point at which a space emerges between ourselves and our pain and distress. Instead of being caught outside in the middle of a thunderstorm, we realise we are watching the thunderstorm through a window, from the safety of our living room.

A research study by Thorsten Barnhofer and colleagues found that mindfulness meditation can be directly helpful in enabling people like Frances to stay alive, because it uncouples the common link between depressive symptoms and suicidal thinking. They followed 194 people with a previous history of suicidal ideas or actions, of whom 77 received a course of mindfulness-based cognitive therapy. When compared with those who had received other forms of psychotherapy, they found significantly fewer suicidal cognitions, even when overall levels of depression remained similar. The conclusion is that mindfulness meditation allows us to decentre from negative thinking, that is to say, it allows us to observe our thoughts and feelings as temporary, objective events in the mind, as opposed to reflections of our selves or our lives that are necessarily true.[44]

I discuss all this with Frances. She says that as a younger woman, brought up in the Catholic tradition, she often used the rosary – a set of prayers accompanied by a strong of knots or beads – as a form of meditation. She tells me she will reflect on whether practicing mindfulness might help her to gain the sense of safety and peace that she has rarely experienced, but that she still believes God intends her to find.

Can Something, Hope

But when we next meet, Frances is in a desperate state. Following a major civil service restructure, she's been informed she will be made redundant at very short notice. And her beloved cat Danny has developed severe, possibly life-threatening kidney problems. Two of her life-supports are under extreme threat. Her hold on life is suddenly in peril. She tells me she does not know whether it is worth keeping going, especially if Danny dies. She is very worried about herself – and so am I. Surely now is the time for me to stop indulging in esoteric discussions about nineteenth-century poetics, and arrange an urgent referral for her to our local mental health team.

And yet, it turns out that Gerard Manley Hopkins can be of immediate service here too. In 'Carrion Comfort', he confronts the question of suicide head on. Should he succumb to his overwhelming despair, when all habitual supports have disappeared, when suicide is a very real and highly attractive option?

His answer, in the first quatrain of the sonnet, is a defiant, magnificent, multiply repeated 'not'.

> Not, I'll not, carrion comfort, Despair, not feast on thee;
> Not untwist — slack they may be — these last strands of man
> In me ór, most weary, cry *I can no more.* I can;
> Can something, hope, wish day come, not choose not to be.

For me, these six 'nots' get right to the heart of the dilemma of existence, and provide the most powerful possible response. Hopkins is treating his despair with the utmost seriousness, even giving it capitalisation and in effect its own persona, but he not going to wallow in it or be defeated by it. He is not going to let anyone or anything feast on his rotting remains. He is not going to allow these last strands of man (the helices of his DNA?) to be unwound. Unlike John Henry Newman's Gerontius, however weary he may be, he is not going to admit defeat and to cry *I can no more*, as he watches his life ebb away.[45] Unlike Hamlet's indecisive 'to be or not to be', and unlike Keats 'half in love with easeful Death' in 'Ode to a Nightingale', Hopkins gives us his emphatic double negative: he can 'not choose not to be'. He is much closer here to the four negatives of the first line of Keats' 'Ode to Melancholy': 'No, No go not to Lethe, neither twist [...]'.[46] Hopkins can. He can stay alive. He can hope.

For Hilary Pearson, this opening quatrain of the sonnet is Hopkins' 'cry of desperate refusal to surrender to the darkness pressing in on him'.[47] I see his refusal to surrender not as a cry of desperation, but as an act of defiance. For me these lines are all about his dogged determination to keep going, come what may.

They resonate, as we will see in Chapter 5, with Al Alvarez' decision to just get on with the business of living; with Stevie Smith (and my mother) resisting suicide in favour of endurance; and perhaps with Peter Porter's injunction to play. They resonate with the mountaineer Joe Simpson, trapped with a fractured tibia on an ice bridge inside a vast crevasse in the Peruvian Andes, faced between the choice of falling into oblivion or trying to find a way out:

> There was no escape upwards, and the drop on the other side was nothing more than an invitation to end it all quickly. I had been tempted, but even in my despair I found I didn't have the courage for suicide. It would be a long time before cold and exhaustion overtook me on the ice bridge, and the idea of waiting alone and maddened for so long had forced me to this choice: abseil until I could find a way out, or die in the process. I would meet it rather than wait for it to come to me.[48]

They resonate too, as we shall see in Chapter 6, with Spinoza's concept of *conatus*: the assumption that we have an innate desire for survival; the belief that 'Each thing, in so far as it is in itself, endeavours to persevere in its being.'[49] As Joshua Hall expresses it

> In these lines, one finds a powerful existential weariness and a counter-force of rugged tenacity fighting to overcome that despair. [...] The poem intertwines both of these aspects, revealing a connection between the essence/conatus of the reader, the speaker of the poem, the author of the poem and by implication human beings in general.[50]

And they resonate, strongly, with Frances. I offer her this sonnet with some trepidation, but she latches eagerly onto these opening lines. She tells me that she can draw immense strength from them, that they encourage her 'to find a steely determination to face my future, whatever it may bring'. She will plod onwards, figuratively and literally: she takes up early morning or late evening walking, often covering several miles of our city streets. My plans for a psychiatric referral can be put on hold, at least for a while.

There is a lot more to 'Carrion Comfort' than this opening quatrain. Over the next four lines, Hopkins launches into a fierce, angry interrogation, demanding to know why he is being treated so appallingly:

> But ah, but O thou terrible, why wouldst thou rude on me
> Thy wring-world right foot rock? lay a lionlimb against me? scan
> With darksome devouring eyes my bruisèd bones? and fan,
> O in turns of tempest, me heaped there; me frantic to avoid thee and flee?

In line six, 'rock' is used as a verb, as in 'why are you rocking me so rudely or roughly with your world-wringing right foot?'. (An earlier draft of these lines read 'Yet why wouldst thou rock rude on me/Thy wring-earth tread.'). A question here is, who is the 'terrible' that Hopkins is addressing? The 'lionlimb' whose dark eyes devour his bruised bones may be the Lion of Judah, in reference to Jesus in the Book of Revelation. Intriguingly, it may also be the devil, in reference to the apostle Peter's first letter where he exhorts his readers to 'Be sober, be vigilant; because your adversary the devil, as a roaring lion, walketh about, seeking whom he may devour'.[51,52] Either way, we are back to God again in line eight, with likely reference to the story of Jonah, heaped up the beach, frantic to avoid him and flee.

Hopkins starts the final sestet with an apparently clear answer to his questions:

Why? That my chaff might fly; my grain lie, sheer and clear.
Nay in all that toil, that coil, since (seems) I kissed the rod,
Hand rather, my heart lo! lapped strength, stole joy, would laugh,
    chéer.

All these trials and tribulations since he 'kissed the rod' (a metaphor for taking holy orders, his ordination as a priest) are there for a purpose, for purification: to strip away the 'chaff', the rubbish that surrounds him, so that his 'grain', his inner being, lies 'sheer and clear'. His strength may have been sapped and his joy stolen, but he can still laugh and cheer.

But then another question presents itself to him. Who, exactly, should he be cheering?

Cheer whom though? the hero whose heaven-handling flung me, fóot
    trod/
Me? or me that fought him? O which one? is it each one? That night,
    that year
Of now done darkness I wretch lay wrestling with (my God!)
    my God.[53]

Whose side should he be taking in this cosmic competition? God's, or his own, or even both? There is direct allusion here to the story in the book of Genesis, with Jacob wrestling all night with a stranger on the banks of a river, eventually realising that the stranger is God, and his relieved conclusion 'I have seen God face to face, and my life is preserved.'[54] Though for Hopkins the struggle has lasted not just a night, but a year. His parenthetic (my God!) remains ambiguous: perhaps an expression of astonishment that he was taking on such a powerful opponent; perhaps an empathic reference to the 'Eli, Eli, Lema Sabaktanei?' That is 'My God, my God, why hast thou forsaken me'[55] of Jesus on the cross.

There are indications that Hopkins is coming through the worst of his torments. Technically, he has a sufficient degree of detachment to experiment with his sonnet structure, using sprung rhythm and a set of 'outrides', with six stressed syllables per line (Whý? That my cháff might flý; my gráin lie, shéer and clear) rather than the standard five. And we have a clue in the last line that the worst is over, as 'of now done darkness' shifts these experiences from present to past tense.

I discuss the second quatrain and the sestet with Frances. Even she, with her Catholic background, finds them a challenge. She is far from convinced that there is some divine purpose behind her redundancy and the likely death of her cat. She smiles sardonically at the implication that these events may be intended for the purification of her soul: arbitrary twists of fate seem more likely to her. She can, however, see something potentially useful in Hopkins' wrestling imagery. It reminds her of two stories from Greek mythology, Achilles' duel with the river-god Scamander, and Menelaus wrestling with the sea-god Proteus. And it reminds me of William Ernest Henley's 'Invictus', his soul 'unconquerable', his head 'bloody but unbowed': 'I am the master of my fate/ I am the captain of my soul'.[56] We agree what all these texts have in common. It is not a question of giving up and meekly accepting our fate. It's the chance to find out that we are strong: stronger than we imagined; strong enough to grapple with the toughest problem life throws at us, and remain undefeated.

Leave Comfort Root-Room

With the fifth and sixth sonnets of this set, we find Hopkins sailing in calmer waters, though he still has a few rocky outcrops to negotiate.

In his sonnet on 'Patience', reverting to his standard iambic pentameters, he begins with the difficult and unattractive qualities of this supposed virtue:

Patience, hard thing! the hard thing but to pray,
But bid for, Patience is! Patience who asks
Wants war, wants wounds; weary his times, his tasks;
To do without, take tosses, and obey.

Although his wrestling is over, he now misses it. There is nothing worthwhile going on. He would rather be at war (he uses 'wants' in line three in the sense of 'lacks' or 'desires') with its risk of wounds, than face the weary monotony of his mundane, daily tasks. We can imagine him feeling a sense of weary resignation at the prospect of having to get back to marking all those tedious undergraduate essays produced by his Classics students at University College. He needs to bid (pray) for patience to get through.

In the second quatrain he introduces the image of ivy to reflect the virtues of patience

> Rare patience roots in these, and, these away,
> Nowhere. Natural heart's ivy, Patience masks
> Our ruins of wrecked past purpose. There she basks
> Purple eyes and seas of liquid leaves all day.

Like ivy, patience grasps, climbs and grows over other surfaces, covering up 'our ruins of wrecked past purpose', hiding our lost ambitions, all those things in our lives that have gone wrong. Its berries and leaves mask the imperfections in a wall, making it appear beautiful, though the underlying problems may still remain. The 'purple eyes' suggest bruises, and the seas of liquid leaves pick up the sense of ruin and wreck in the previous line, suggesting that 'Natural heart's ivy' is 'a kind of limpet, coraling the shipwrecked heart'.[57]

In the sestet Hopkins compares the natural man and the virtuous man, now changing his imagery from ivy to honeycombs.

> We hear our hearts grate on themselves: it kills
> To bruise them dearer. Yet the rebellious wills
> Of us we do bid God bend to him even so.
> And where is he who more and more distils
> Delicious kindness? - He is patient. Patience fills
> His crisp combs, and that comes those ways we know.[58]

He brings the heart into the conversation, but now he is talking about hearts in general, rather than to his own as in 'I Wake and Feel'. His argument here is a strongly Christian one: man on his own can only cover over the wreck of his past purposes. The ivy risks causing further damage to the underlying structures, 'it kills to bruise them dearer'. But only with divine intervention can the empty space be transformed by 'delicious kindness', producing 'crisp combs' of honey.

These last three lines clearly strike a chord with Frances, who says 'that last bit makes a lot of sense to me', but they leave me less satisfied. While I can enjoy and see the purpose of Hopkins' metaphoric change from ivy to honey, I do not believe that we need divine intervention to achieve lasting inner peace. Frances and I agree to disagree, and we move on to the final sonnet of this set, 'My own heart', with its emphasis on care and kindness to the self in times of trouble. This is one of my all-time favourite poems, and here it is in full.

> My own heart let me more have pity on; let
> Me live to my sad self hereafter kind,
> Charitable; not live this tormented mind
> With this tormented mind tormenting yet.
> I cast for comfort I can no more get
> By groping round my comfortless, than blind
> Eyes in their dark can day or thirst can find
> Thirst's all-in-all in all a world of wet.
>
> Soul, self; come, poor Jackself, I do advise
> You, jaded, let be; call off thoughts awhile
> Elsewhere; leave comfort root-room; let joy size
> At God knows when to God knows what; whose smile
> 's not wrung, see you; unforeseen times rather — as skies
> Betweenpie mountains — lights a lovely mile.[59]

There is an expanding sense of interior space as this poem progresses, a feeling of having (at long last) found a little room to rest, to breathe, to grow. Hopkins is back in dialogue with his heart, now as its guide and protector. He is beginning to be gentler with his 'sad self', giving himself a break from his incessant internal critical chatter. It's time to stop the endless tormenting cycles of tormenting his tormented mind and 'call off thoughts awhile elsewhere'. His world may still be comfortless and dark, but he is beginning to have a sense of control over his life, and an awareness that his 'Jackself', though he may be common and master of nothing, deserves kindness and love. He can practice self-compassion.

We can be compassionate to ourselves – have pity on our hearts – just as much as we are towards others. We can treat ourselves just as well as we treat our friends and the people we love. For Kristin Neff, self-compassion has three basic elements. Self-kindness, in place of self-judgement, means 'being warm and understanding toward ourselves when we suffer, fail or feel inadequate, rather than ignoring our pain or flagellating ourselves with self-criticism'.[60] Awareness of our common humanity in place of isolation, means recognising that suffering and a sense of personal inadequacy are part of the shared human experience. And mindfulness, observing rather than identifying with our negative thoughts, allowing our feelings and emotions to be neither suppressed nor exaggerated.

Robin Hardwick-Smith pursued a successful career as a family doctor in New Zealand. He found himself increasingly frustrated by the limitations of what medicine had to offer his patients, and progressively more aware of his inability to care for himself and to form genuine close relationships with other people. In his biography he explains how neither alcohol nor suicidal solo sailing adventures addressed his increasingly desperate sense of frustration. Instead, through meditation practice he found compassion:

> a universal quality that pervades all [....] the ordinary response, to suffering, of a self-accepting, self-loving being wherever it manifests – including within myself.[61]

Frances and I discuss how she can do the same. She can challenge her negative thoughts. She can take time out from tormenting herself about why she feels so unhappy. She can stop yelling 'Just pull yourself together, stupid' inside her own head. She can recognise her own worth, realise that it's alright to feel the way she does. I now feel comfortable about exploring mindfulness meditation with her again. I tell her about the results of a recent randomised controlled trial of mindfulness-based compassionate living, where the focus is on developing compassion towards oneself as well as the world around. This trial showed significant benefits, including reduction in thoughts of suicide and self-harm, for a group of people like her with experience of severe, prolonged, recurrent depressive symptoms.[62] She decides it is well worth a go, perhaps incorporating it into her early morning walking routines.

I love Hopkins' phrase 'leave comfort root-room'. It's about giving ourselves permission and space for a sense of ease and well-being to set down roots and begin to grow. And then, who knows, joy may (increase in) size and catch us unawares. Hopkins' evocative image of God's smile, distilled within his new word 'betweenpie', is of a brightly dappled sky seen between dark mountains. For him that may well bring back memories of the hills of north Wales during his happier times in the seminary there. For me it conjures up childhood days of sunshine and cloud over Glendalough in County Wicklow, Ireland.

We can help that joyful smile to grow. One way that works for me is the meditation technique of visualising a constant, infinite stream of warm, spacious, liquid sunshine; pouring in through the top of my head; slowly and gradually filling my body, from my toes all the way upwards.

Plough Down Sillion Shine

From here it is a small step to rekindle our compassion for others, returning in our imagination with Hopkins as he undertakes one of his palliative care visits to Felix Randal in his Liverpool parish. Recognising that we ourselves receive comfort and a greater sense of well-being as we provide comfort to others; that we feel, we become, more appreciated and more loved.

And then, if we are fortunate, we catch the occasional, unforeseen glimpse of unalloyed delight. On a clear, sunny, spring day like today, writing in my study, overlooking my garden as it bursts with blossom from apple, cherry, pear and plum trees, I find myself effortlessly travelling back in time with Hopkins, together leaving our cares behind as we revisit his ecstatic vision of 'The Windhover', early on the morning of 30 May 1877 in the countryside of north Wales.

> I caught this morning morning's minion, king-
> dom of daylight's dauphin, dapple-dawn-drawn Falcon, in his riding
> Of the rolling level underneath him steady air, and striding
> High there, how he rung upon the rein of a wimpling wing
> In his ecstasy! then off, off forth on swing,
> As a skate's heel sweeps smooth on a bow-bend: the hurl and gliding
> Rebuffed the big wind. My heart in hiding
> Stirred for a bird, – the achieve of, the mastery of the thing!
>
> Brute beauty and valour and act, oh, air, pride, plume, here
> Buckle! AND the fire that breaks from thee then, a billion
> Times told lovelier, more dangerous, O my chevalier!
>
> No wonder of it: shéer plód makes plough down sillion
> Shine, and blue-bleak embers, ah my dear,
> Fall, gall themselves, and gash gold-vermilion[63].

This sonnet works best when read aloud. It takes a few goes to get the rhythm of it, especially the first few lines. Do try it yourself. You'll soon find you are flying with the falcon, up and down, barely taking a breath until the first full stop arrives, half way though line seven.

Then have a rest and check out some of the words and images. In line two 'dauphin' means 'crown prince', and for Hopkins offers direct linkage with Jesus. In line six the imagery is of ice-skating: for us it could as easily be of a post-pandemic skiing holiday in the Alps, or surfing the waves of Cornwall. The sestet begins with the image of the crown prince on horseback fastening (buckling) together his armour. 'Plough down sillion shine' refers to the way that soil, when turned over by a plough, gleams in the sunshine. In the final line, 'gall' means graze or scrape, and 'gold-vermilion' is the colour both of fire and of freshly spilt blood.

Hopkins' concept of inscape, the charged essence of a thing, its sanctity, its uniqueness and purpose in the world, applies in abundance to the falcon. His related concept instress, the energy that holds the thing together and the impulse which carries it whole into the mind of the person seeing it, is also fully realised here. His heart (and mine) stirs for the bird. We are at one with it in its mastery of the air.

As I have observed before, we do not need to share Hopkins' religious convictions to gain profound hope from this sonnet. The beauty and joy of the falcon, ecstatically riding the wind, infuses with his energy not only Hopkins the poet but also ourselves the readers. He reminds us to celebrate those – perhaps fleeting – moments in our own lives when we feel effortlessly magnificent and free. He inspires us to believe in a glittering luminous core to our own being, a core not suppressed by our daily strivings but rather brought by them to the surface, honed and sparkling in the sun. And all this is in full awareness that our existence is ephemeral and contingent, that danger and death await us; which knowledge serves only to heighten the intensity of our life in the present moment.[64]

Notes

1 Gerard Manley Hopkins, 'No Worst, There is None', *The Poems Gerard Manley Hopkins*, ed. Robert Bridges (London: Humphrey Milford, 1918), no. 41.

2 Piotr Tchaikovsky, 'Adagio lamentoso' *Symphonie No 6 Pathetique*, Orchestra del Teatro alla Scala of Milan, dir. Yuri Temirkanov, accessed 27 March 2021. https://www.youtube.com/watch?v=BGIL_yyT3wI.

3 Christopher Dowrick C. 'Comfort in a Whirlwind: Literature and Distress in General Practice', in *Reading and Mental Health*, ed. Josie Billington (Cham, Switzerland: Palgrave Macmillan, 2019), 15–30.

4 Christopher Dowrick, 'From Despair to Delight: a journey of six sonnets', http://wellbecoming.blogspot.com/ posts 2 to 15 April 2018, (accessed 27 March 2021).

5 Anthony Domestico, 'Inscape, instress and distress', *Commonweal* (2009), 9 March. Accessed 29 March 2021. https://www.commonwealmagazine.org/inscape-instress-distress?_ga=1.190997742.596395981.1472016212.

6 Hopkins, 'Journal entry 12 December 1872', in William Gardner (ed.), *Poems and Prose of Gerard Manley Hopkins* (London, Penguin, 1968), 127.

7 Hopkins, 'Letter to Canon Richard Watson Dixon', quoted in Paul Mariani, *Gerard Manley Hopkins: A Life* (New York: Viking, 2008), 263.

8 Simon Szreter and Graham Mooney, 'Urbanization Mortality and the Standard of Living Debate: New Estimates of the Expectation of Life at Birth in Nineteenth-Century British Cities' *Economic History Review* 51, no. 1 (1998): 84–112.

9 Hopkins, 'Felix Randal', in Bridges, *Hopkins*, ibid., no. 29.

10 Hopkins, 'Letter to Baillie', quoted in Mariani, *Hopkins*, ibid., 348.

11 Hopkins, 'Letter to Robert Bridges', in Gardner, *Hopkins*, ibid., 202.

12 Norman White, 'Review of *Inspirations Unbidden* by Daniel Harris', *The Hopkins Quarterly*, 11, no. 3–4, (1985): 87–96 (89).

13 The original letter has 'three' crossed out, with 'four' added instead. William Gardner notes (ibid., 240) that these four are probably 'To Seem the Stranger', 'I Wake and Feel', 'Patience' and 'My Own Heart'. The other is 'Ash Boughs'.

14 Hopkins, 'Letter to Robert Bridges 1 September 1885', quoted in Mariani, *Hopkins*, ibid., 357–58.

15 Nic Roark, 'Gerard Manley Hopkins and a Spirituality of Despair'. Accessed 29 March 2021. www.academia.edu/5050232/Gerard_Manley_Hopkins_and_a_ Spirituality_of_Despair.

16 Daniel Harris, *Inspirations Unbidden: The 'Terrible Sonnets' of Gerard Manley Hopkins*. (Berkeley: University of California Press, 1982), xv.

17 J Hillis Miller, *The Disappearance of God: Five Nineteenth-Century Writers* (New York: Schoken Books, 1965), 352–53.

18 White, 'Review of Harris', ibid., 87–96.

19 Mariani, *Hopkins*, ibid.

20 Paul Mariani. *A Commentary on the Complete Poems of Gerard Manley Hopkins* (New York: Cornell University Press, 1970), 12.

21 Sørina Higgins and Rebecca Tirrell Talbot, 'Between Two Strange Hearts: Spiritual Desolation in the Later Poetry of Gerard Manley Hopkins & Charles Williams'. *Inklings Forever* 8 (2012): 1–10.

22 Maria Lichtmann, 'Gerard Manley Hopkins: Contemplative Hero', *Spiritus: A Journal of Christian Spirituality* 1 (2001): 172–85.

23 Hopkins, 'Patience', in Bridges, *Hopkins*, ibid, no. 44.

24 Emile Durkheim, *Suicide: A Study in Sociology*, trans. John Spaulding and George Simpson (London: Routledge, 2005).

25 Karl Marx, *The Economic and Philosophic Manuscripts of 1844*, trans. Martin Milligan, (New York: International Publishers, 1964).

26 Anna Mueller et al., 'The Social Roots of Suicide: Theorizing How the External Social World Matters to Suicide and Suicide Prevention'. *Frontiers in Psychology* 12 (2021): 621569.

27 Jie Zhang, 'The Strain Theory of Suicide'. *Journal of Pacific Rim Psychology* 13 (2019): e27.

28 Harris, *Inspirations Unbidden*, ibid., 124.

29 Matthew Carbery, 'Exiled in Dublin: Gerard Manley Hopkins and John Berryman', paper to Plymouth Landscapes conference (2013). Accessed 1 April 2021. www. academia.edu/13049620/Exiled_In_Dublin_Gerard_Manley_Hopkins_and_ John_Berryman.

30 *Christian Bible, King James Version* (KJV): Lamentations 3:8.

31 *KJV*: Psalm 88:18.

32 Thomas Joiner. *Why People Die By Suicide* (Cambridge, MA, US: Harvard University Press; 2005).

33 Johanna Lynch, *A Whole Person Approach to Wellbeing: Building a Sense of Safety* (Abingdon: Routledge, 2021).

34 Harris, *Inspirations Unbidden*, ibid., 52.

35 Rory O'Connor. 'Towards an Integrated Motivational–Volitional Model of Suicidal Behaviour'. In Rory O'Connor et al. eds. *International Handbook of Suicide Prevention: Research, Policy and Practice* (Chichester, UK: Wiley, 2001), 181–98.

36 Mariani, *Hopkins*, ibid., 340.

37 Jean Paul Sartre, *Sketch for a Theory of the Emotions*, trans. Philip Mairet (London: Routledge, 1971), 70.

38 Hopkins, 'I Wake and feel', in Bridges, *Hopkins*, ibid., no. 45.

39 Jean Paul Sartre, *Nausea*, trans. Lloyd Alexander L (New York: New Directions, 1964), 34.

40 *KJV,* Job 38:1–4.

41 Mariani, *Hopkins,* ibid., 346.

42 Brett Beasley, 'Hopkins's Approach to Mortality and His Innovations in Poetic Form'. *The Hopkins Quarterly* 41, (2014): 79–99.

43 See for example: https://www.headspace.com/mindfulness [accessed 25 July 2021].

44 Thorsten Barnhofer et al., 'Mindfulness-Based Cognitive Therapy (MBCT) Reduces the Association between Depressive Symptoms and Suicidal Cognitions in Patients With a History of Suicidal Depression'. *Journal of Consulting and Clinical Psychology* 83, no. 6 (2015): 1013–20.

45 Quotation from John Henry Newman, *The Dream of Gerontius,* ed. Julius Gliebe (New York: Schwartz, Kirwin & Fauss, 1916), in Beasley, 'Hopkins' approach', ibid., 85.

46 John Keats, *Selected Poems,* (London: Penguin Classics, 2007).

47 Hilary Pearson, 'The Terrible Sonnets of Gerard Manley Hopkins and the spirituality of depression'. *The Way,* 46, no. 1 (2007): 23–37.

48 Joe Simpson, *Touching the Void* (New York: Vintage Books, 1998), 130.

49 Baruch Spinoza, *Ethics,* ed. and trans. George Parkinson (Oxford: Oxford University Press, 2000), part III proposition 6.

50 Joshua Hall, 'Poetic intuition: Spinoza and Gerard Manley Hopkins'. *Philosophy Today* 57 (2013): 401–07.

51 *KJV, 1 Peter 5:8.*

52 Alan Rose, 'Hopkins' "Carrion Comfort": The Artful Disorder of Prayer'. *Victorian Poetry* 15, no. 3, (1977): 207–17.

53 Hopkins, 'Carrion Comfort', in Bridges, *Hopkins,* ibid., no. 40.

54 *KJV,* Genesis 32:40.

55 *KJV,* Psalm 22:1 and Matthew 27:46.

56 William Henley, 'Invictus', *A Book of Verses* (New York: Scribner & Welford. 1891), 56–57.

57 John Glavin, '"The Exercise of Saints": Hopkins, Milton, and Patience'. *Texas Studies in Literature and Language* 20, no. 2, (1978): 139–52.

58 Hopkins, 'Patience', in Bridges, *Hopkins,* ibid., no. 46.

59 Hopkins, 'My Own Heart', in Bridges, *Hopkins,* ibid., no. 47.

60 Kristin Neff, 'Self-Compassion'. Accessed 9 April 2021. https://self-compassion.org/the-three-elements-of-self-compassion-2/.

61 Taranatha. *Steps to Happiness: Travelling from Depression and Addiction to the Buddhist Path* (Birmingham: Windhorse Publications, 2006), 96.

62 Rhoda Schuling et al., 'Recovery from Recurrent Depression: Randomized Controlled Trial of the Efficacy of Mindfulness-Based Compassionate Living Compared with Treatment-As-Usual on Depressive Symptoms and Its Consolidation at Longer Term Follow-Up'. *Journal of Affective Disorders* 273 (2020): 265–73.

63 Hopkins, 'The Windhover', in Bridges, *Hopkins,* ibid., no. 12.

64 Dowrick, in *Reading and Mental Health,* Billington, ibid., 28.

Chapter 5

POINTS OF TRANSFORMATION

Sorrow is my own yard
where the new grass
flames as it has flamed
often before but not
with the cold fire
that closes round me this year.
Thirty five years
I lived with my husband.
The plumtree is white today
with masses of flowers.
Masses of flowers
load the cherry branches
and color some bushes
yellow and some red
but the grief in my heart
is stronger than they
for though they were my joy
formerly, today I notice them
and turn away forgetting.
Today my son told me
that in the meadows,
at the edge of the heavy woods
in the distance, he saw
trees of white flowers.
I feel that I would like
to go there
and fall into those flowers
and sink into the marsh near them.[1]

I now switch my gaze from the particular to the general. In this chapter, I explore the ways in which literary texts may act as points of transformation in the face of the grief, loss and despair so eloquently expression in this poem by William Carlos Williams. Having considered in detail how Leo Tolstoy and Gerard Manley Hopkins each wrestled with the dilemma of their existence, including their profound though radically differing religious experiences, I broaden my horizons to reflect on themes and perspectives that have emerged from my own reading over the past five decades, with the help of some contemporary literary criticism.

Starting with James Joyce's portrayal of suicide as an everyday temptation, I discuss Al Alvarez's ambivalence towards the act and his conclusion that it is nothing more than a denial of experience. With Peter Porter, I reflect on the cost of seriousness and consider what other options there may be for us when life seems too difficult to continue: perhaps the gritty endurance of Stevie Smith and my mother; perhaps the political awareness of Zbigniew Herbert and Seamus Heaney; or perhaps the creative fiction of Nick Hornby and Matt Haig. With reference to David Foster Wallace and my patient Leigh, I discuss the inexplicability of suicide to those bereft by it and consider – with the help of Graham Swift and Maggie O'Farrell – how new ways of living may emerge for those who are left behind. And finally, travelling back in time from north London in the twenty-first century through tenth-century Iceland to ancient Egypt, I show how support from those close to us – or from people we meet by accident – can make the difference between death and life.

An Everyday Temptation

Episodes of suicide appear in almost all James Joyce's works, portrayed simultaneously as both tragic and banal. Joyce is so open to experience that he is interested in exploring these two extremes, as well as points between. He presents the paradox that suicide can be seen as an act that is both ultimately meaningful, and yet trivial, contingent, and quotidian.

In *Portrait of the Artist as a Young Man*, Joyce is obsessed with falling – or failing. The suicidality of overreaching ambition is epitomised in the conflation of Dedalus with his son Icarus flying too close to the sun at the very end of the novel.

Dubliners has two suicides amongst its stories. In circumstances deliberately reminiscent of Anna Karenina,[2] Joyce presents the 'painful case' of Mrs Emily Simico, knocked down and killed by the ten o'clock slow train from Kingstown, her life having disintegrated after an unrequited love affair with Mr James Duffy. In *The Dead* (my favourite amongst all the wonders of Joyce's writings) we have Michael Furey killing himself for love of Gretta – 'I think he died for me' – and a suicidal meaning within Gabriel's final response to his wife's confession. 'The time had come for him to set out on his journey westward' refers not only his desire to change from being a West Briton and espouse Irish nationalism but also to the notion of re-enacting his wife's lover's suicide, taking a journey to the west, understood as the land of the dead:

> His soul swooned slowly as he heard the snow falling faintly through the universe and faintly falling, like the descent of their last end, upon all the living and the dead.[3]

Suicide is permanently on Leopold Bloom's mind throughout *Ulysses*. He refers to it explicitly 11 times during the day (16 June 1904) in Dublin on which the story takes place, mainly in relation to memories of his father Rudolph's suicide 18 years previously. While riding in a carriage to attend Paddy Dignam's funeral, for example, he has to endure this conversation between his two companions, only one of whom knows the story about his father's death.

> -But the worst of it all, Mr Power said, is the man who takes his own life.
> Martin Cunningham drew out his watch briskly, coughed and put it back.
> -The greatest disgrace to have in the family, Mr Power added.
> -Temporary insanity, of course, Martin Cunningham said decisively.
>   We must take a charitable view of it.
> -They say a man who does it is a coward, Mr Dedalus said.
> -It is not for us to judge, Martin Cunningham said.
> Mr Bloom, about to speak, closed his lips again. Martin Cunningham's
>   large eyes. Looking away now. Sympathetic human man he is [...]
> He looked away from me. He knows.

Bloom cannot find a way to contribute to this discussion. The emotions it evoke are too complex and still, after all this time, too raw. But it brings memories flooding back to him:

> That afternoon of the inquest. The redlabelled bottle on the table. The room in the hotel with the hunting pictures. Stuffy it was, Sunlight through the slats of the Venetian blinds. The coroner's ears, big and hairy. Boots giving evidence. Thought he was asleep first. Then saw like yellow streaks on his face. Had slipped down to the foot of the bed. Verdict: overdose. Death by misadventure. The letter. For my son Leopold.

> No more pain. Wake no more. Nobody owns.[4]

No more pain for his father perhaps, his death an end to his own suffering, but still a heavy burden for Bloom to carry: he keeps his father's suicide letter, addressed *To My Dear Son Leopold* and filled with a sense of unbearable longing for his dead wife, in a locked drawer at his home.

It is not coincidental that Joyce considered his own father John a potential suicide. Bloom takes his father's penname Virag (Hungarian for Flower) when he writes to his lover. And at different times both Stephen Dedalus and Bloom contemplate throwing themselves off the cliffs near Dublin into the sea. Here is Bloom's recollection of himself as a teenager, too ugly for girls to play with him, looking down into the sea from high up on Ben Howth:

> BLOOM: (*Hatless, flushed, covered with burrs of thistledown and gorse-pine*). Regularly engaged. Circumstances alter cases. (*He gazes intently downwards on the water*) Thirtytwo head over heels per second. Sad end of government printer's clerk. (*Through silversilent summer air the dummy of Bloom, rolled in a mummy, rolls rotatingly from the Lion's Head cliff into the purple waiting waters.*)[5]

Ultimately, for Bloom and for Joyce, suicide is 'an everyday temptation',[6] hidden in plain sight because of its simplicity and familiarity. But for all that, it remains a haunting, tragic reminder of the frailty and precarity of our lives.

A Denial of Experience

I first read *Savage God*, Al Alvarez' 1970s review of suicide in literature,[7] just a few years after it was published, initially to find out more about the death of Sylvia Plath. I was in my mid-20s, at least half in love with her, captivated by her obsession with death and disturbed by her turbulent relationship with Ted Hughes whose jaunty, vicious, murderous Crow – pure death instinct – I also, confusingly, admired. My own marriage was crumbling, I was increasingly doubtful about my religious faith and frustrated with my chosen career in social work.

Alvarez not only answered my questions about Plath, but also introduced me to a whole new world, which struck me as risky and dangerous but yet, at the same time, fascinating, exciting and even seductive. Coming back to *Savage God* now I still see the risk and dangers, but no longer the excitement: instead what I find now are Alvarez' courage and compassion. And, at the very end of the book, in light of his own experience as a 'failed suicide', he offers me my second point of transformation.

Alvarez doesn't believe in solutions, since suicide means different things to different people at different times. His aim is rather to explore the 'shabby, confused, agonised crisis which is the common reality of suicide' and, in so doing to counterbalance two prevailing currents of thought: the religious prejudice against suicide as high crime, and the scientific denial of 'all serious meaning by reducing despair to the boniest statistics'.

His discussion of Plath's last months and weeks remains compelling and authoritative, based on his personal friendship with her, and his sense that he let her down at a time of great need, when separation from Ted Hughes resurrected her grief for her father. He is confident that she did not intend to die, but was making one last desperate attempt to exorcise death (and her father). A letter to her therapist went astray. She left her children asleep upstairs, confident that the au pair would find them and her when she arrived in the morning; but there was a problem with the lock and the au pair couldn't get through front door.

He writes movingly about severe depression as a 'spiritual winter, frozen, sterile, unmoving', and the irresistible internal logic of suicidal thought, generating 'a shut off, impregnable but wholly convincing world where every detail fits and each incident reinforces his decision'. He is strongly influenced by Freud's theories of mourning and melancholia which I discussed in Chapter 2, where (like Plath and her father, or John Donne and his mistress) the mourner sets up the lost object in their own ego, but the consequent guilt and hostility become too much to bear. He wonders if Freud's death instinct is not so much to do with primary aggression as primary pessimism, and notes Philip Larkin's view that 'Beneath it all, desire for oblivion runs'.

He then embarks on a dazzling exposition of suicide in (primarily European) literature, from Dante's seventh circle of hell – a dark pathless wood where souls of suicides grow as warped poisonous thorns – through the more sympathetic understandings of John Donne and Robert Burton, and on into the romantic agonies of Thomas Chatterton, John Keats and Percy Bysshe Shelley, for whom creativity was the preserve of the young, where once again we find Goethe's *Werther*, martyr to unrequited love and excessive sensibility.

By the twentieth century, Alvarez notes, suicide is 'something people do, like adultery'. As with Joyce, it has become a normalised activity. With the fragmentation of values, and the moral bankruptcy of the world after the First World War, the 'new permanent condition of the arts was depression'. Life is an art object, but worthless. Wilfred Owen's letters to his mother describe the numbness of soldiers 'more terrible than terror, for it was a blindfold look, and without expression, like a dead rabbit's'.[8] For Alvarez, this psychic numbing in the face of overwhelming death 'is the final quantum to which all modish forms of twentieth-century alienation are reduced'.

In the final pages of *Savage God*, Alvarez describes his own highly dangerous but ultimately unsuccessful attempt to take his own life. He calls this his 'dismal confession', and appears somewhat embarrassed as he relates how recurrent depressive episodes stemming back to childhood and parental example (both his parents reportedly thought putting one's head in the gas oven was a perfectly natural thing to do), followed by a difficult marriage where arguments were both fuelled and resolved by alcohol, led him one Christmas to the inevitable conclusion that he must end it all by consuming his secret stash of 45 tablets. Unlike Sylvia Plath, his wife found him in time and he was rushed to hospital for resuscitation.

I don't remember paying much attention to this account when I first read it all those decades ago. But now, paradoxically, I find his subsequent response to this episode to be the most hopeful element of the whole book. This is what he says:

> Above all, I was disappointed. Somehow, I felt, death had let me down; I had expected more of it. I had looked for something overwhelming, an experience which would clarify all my confusions. But it turned out simply to be a denial of experience [...] I though death would be [...] a synoptic vision of life, crisis by crisis, all suddenly explained, justified, redeemed, a Last Judgement in the coils and circuits of the brain. Instead all I got was a hole in the head, a round zero, nothing. I'd been swindled.[9]

So, he decided to just get on with living. Once he had realised that death was not going to provide him with any answers – that it was merely 'a denial of experience' – he found that he no longer worried very much about whether he was happy or unhappy. Some glimmers of hope emerge. The problem of problems no longer existed. 'And that in itself was already the beginning of happiness'. Like Albert Camus (of whom a lot more in Chapter 6) he has the realisation that there is 'only one liberty, to come to terms with death'.

Alvarez is studiously careful to avoid judgement towards or offer solutions for others, which makes his personal testimony all the more persuasive. He has come to terms with death. He has recognised its futility, its pointlessness. It no longer offers him any attractions, any sense of fulfilment or achievement. After that, everything in life becomes possible. Even if, sometimes, the life we are able to live may just be a matter of getting through the day as best we can. Just plodding on, putting one foot down on the ground and then the other, literally and imaginatively. We may imagine ourselves joining my patient Frances on one of her early morning walks round the streets of Liverpool, facing the loss of her civil service job and (more importantly) her cat, gradually finding the 'steely determination' to face her future, whatever it may bring.

Just plodding on for a while provides us with the space, and the opportunity, to look at life differently. I now look at some of the ways in which we can do that.

Prate Not to Me of Suicide

Hospitalised for three years from the age of five, with tuberculous peritonitis, Stevie Smith became 'early accustomed to the thought of death by suicide'.

> 'Death is my servant', she wrote 'There is a very deadly poison in the fear that things may become more than we can bear. [...] But with death our immediate ally, such thoughts vanish'.[10]

Circling around Freud's death instinct, for Smith the ever-present option of death breaks the human pattern and frees her from the cares of the world. Suicidal ideation has a calming, restorative effect, expressed most succinctly in her 1957 bilingual poem *The Bottle of Aspirins*. Here, we find her in jocular dialogue with a male presence from the land of suicides, discussing how a couple of hundred aspirins will free them from all distress. We observe Smith's use of splitting throughout this brief poem: the ambiguous use of 'I' and 'him', and the switch between English and French, a language that is familiar to her but emphatically not her own. Displacing thoughts of suicide onto someone else allows her to articulate them in poetry. We have already seen a similar technique at work in Hopkins' *I Wake and Feel*, when he entertains a dialogue between himself and his heart. And the poem reminds me of several patients who I know keep 'emergency packs' of medications which would enable them to end it all if they decided to do so but, at the same time, enables them to keep going precisely because they know that they have a genuine choice in the matter.

As Juliet Stevenson brings out in her outstanding performance in the Dead Poets Live series at Shakespeare's Globe,[11] through her exploration of the cavities of pain, her juxtaposition of desolation and giddiness, Smith displays remarkable courage in the face of despair. Death defines the scope of her immediacy. It is the inspiration that keeps her going.

Smith's insistence on the therapeutic value of the contemplation of death, and suicide in particular, is not uncontested. She provided several different interpretations of her most famous poem – *Not Waving but Drowning* – to the point where Andrew Bennett observes that all we can conclude is that the poem is 'about ways in which language breaks down [...] when it comes to [...] writing poems about suicide'.[12] In later life (she died at age 68 of a brain tumour), she writes of death as 'the sweet prairies of anarchy' but also exhorts us to 'Keep Death where he would be, in his own place'. Although there is a consistency in her sense of romance with death – which she often describes in heroic masculine terms, her poetry reflects a deep ambivalence between the option of bailing out (as in the Bottle of Aspirins) and the sense of having to continue on with life, while longing not to do so.

The sense of having to continue with life is most prominent in her 1942 poem, *Study to Deserve Death*. In this poem, she insists that death is be earned: it must be seen as a worthy achievement, merited only by those who take a warrior-like attitude to life, who never give up and continue to fight their way through to the very end. Suicide has been struck off the agenda. Endurance is the key:

> Prate not to me of suicide,
> Faint heart in battle, not for pride
> I say Endure, but that such end denied
> Makes welcomer yet the death that's to be died.[13]

For me, this poem has multiple meanings. In the direct context of this chapter, the whole poem, especially the line 'prate not to me of suicide', with 'to prate' understood as 'to talk foolishly or at tedious length about something', is a scornful criticism of self-destruction in favour of the Hopkins-like endurance we saw in *Carrion Comfort*, of tackling head on whatever life throws at us, not running away. It may well have been an argument with and against herself, in the context of the second world war and an expression of her need to subsume personal desires in favour of collective effort against a common external threat. As such, it is another potential point of transformation, another opportunity for a different way of looking at our lives in the world.

More specifically it has profound personal meaning, since at my mother's request I read it aloud to hundreds of people during my father's memorial service in Durham Cathedral in December 1987. I remember feeling very uncomfortable about it at the time. My father had served with distinction in the navy during the Second World War, before becoming an academic lawyer, so I could see some straightforward symbolism there. But the suicide references didn't immediately make sense, indeed they grated against my understanding of how he had lived his life. It was some time later that I realised this poem was only superficially about my father. It was primarily a message from my mother, via me, back to herself. It was a public declaration that, no matter how much she longed to die in the hope of being reunited with him – and for many years afterwards this was her foremost, persistent wish – it was her duty to endure, to continue to strive towards the death she would one day long into the future deserve, to remain alive for the sake of her 3 sons, for the sake of her 10 grandchildren, for the sake of her 14 great-grandchildren and for the sake of loving and supporting them all through their joys and despairs, rather than embrace the death she so urgently then desired.

The Artist Must Play

Seriousness in literature does not, in fact, lead inexorably to suicide. William Wootten's critique of *The Alvarez Generation*[14] offers a valuable antidote to the poetics of psychic disturbance. He shows how Alvarez himself rowed back over time from his depiction of poetry as 'a murderous art' to the more nuanced position we find in *Savage God*, and to his later concern about his own complicity in Plath's death, that perhaps 'all our rash chatter about art and risk and courage' may have even 'egged her on'.[15] And he notes Peter Porter's deep concerns that suicide 'has become the endorsement not merely of genius but of seriousness'.[16]

Following the suicide of his wife Jannice, and the death of his fellow poet Veronica Forrest-Thompson, Porter responds with his 1978 poem *The Cost of Seriousness*. In this crucial poem, Porter severs the link between suicide and poetic creativity and excellence. If poetry is the way in which we discover and express our innermost thoughts and feelings, if we find through poetry that life isn't living up to our expectations, if we realise that our creative endeavours are not working out as we wished them to, we do not have to assume that ending it all is the only answer. If the cost of seriousness is death, if taking our words and the world around us too seriously leads us to self-destruct then, he concludes, seriousness has to be avoided:

Which is why the artist must play.[17]

For Porter here, 'play' is proposed as the essential antidote to 'seriousness'. As such it has several possible meanings.

It can be play as a sense of light-heartedness, of enjoyment and fun, even in the face of life's difficulties. Maybe such play takes the form of the gentle poetic ironies of Pam Ayres with her incorrigible husband,[18] or Wisława Szymborska's tales of cats, monkeys and sea cucumbers.[19] Or maybe it takes the form of complete distraction from the seriousness of life, which for me involves various forms of physical exercise (today it was open water swimming in Queen's Dock, Liverpool) or – ideally – five days of a closely contested cricket match between England and India.

But avoidance and distraction are not the only options available. To 'play' also means to take part, to engage in a particular role or activity. In this alternative sense, poetry is more than capable of coping coolly with facts that could easily slide out of control. In post-war eastern Europe we find the Polish poet Zbigniew Herbert enduring and subverting the Soviet totalitarian experiments with razor-sharp irony, most notably in *Damastes (also known as Procrustes) Speaks*. Inventing a bed with the dimensions of the perfect man, Damastes catches unwary travellers and invites them to rest for the night in his inn. In order to make them fit his perfect bed, he has to stretch the limbs of some and cut the legs of others. Inevitably some of his 'patients' died, but the more that did so

> the more I was certain my research was right
> the goal was noble progress requires victims.[20]

Incidentally, in describing the victims as patients, Herbert identifies the brutal Utopian reformer as a doctor. For me, as for Iona Heath,[21] this is a profoundly disturbing thought.

And we find Seamus Heaney, growing up in a Catholic, nationalist community in Derry in Northern Ireland, reflecting on the Troubles, the often-violent political struggles that deeply affected his country during his lifetime. He begins to weave the ongoing conflict into a broader historical frame in his 1975 poetic collection *North* of which the second, shorter part contains poems that deal specifically with life in Northern Ireland during the Troubles. He writes of British Ulster as the ministry of fear, reflects on how Goya's painting 'The Third of May 1808' resonates with the police firing on the inhabitants of the Falls Road in Belfast in the summer of 1969, and describes himself as a wood-kerne, in reference to Irish irregular foot-soldiers of the sixteenth century. In *Two Lorries*, from his 1996 collection *The Spirit Level*, he juxtaposes memories of his childhood life with the more recent troubles, as one lorry cheerfully delivering coal to his mother's home is followed by another, filled with bombs, about to reduce a local bus station to dust and ashes.

Seriousness and play do not have to be dichotomous, polar opposites. We have the Buddhist concept of 'serious playfulness', the combination of concern and humility which enables us to be both involved and carefree at the same time. It is possible to play with seriousness, not with the bleak gallows humour of Plath, but in ways that offer the prospect of change and even hope.

Nick Hornby and Matt Haig provide strong, contrasting examples of how to do this.

In Nick Hornby's darkly comedic *A Long Way Down*, four deeply unhappy people – Martin, a disgraced television presenter, Maureen, single parent of a child with disabilities, Jess, an irritable and irritating teenager, and failed rock star JJ – all decide to kill themselves on New Year's Eve. They each have the intention to jump from the roof of 'Toppers' House', a north London tower-block with a reputation for self-destruction. But their plans are ruined when they meet each other on the roof. Killing oneself in peaceful, reflective solitude is one thing; doing so in front of others is quite another: far too embarrassing and besides, what is the etiquette about who jumps first? As Martin puts it:

> Why it didn't occur to us that a well-known suicide spot would be like Piccadilly Circus on New Year's Eve I have no idea, but at that point in the proceedings I had accepted the reality of our situation: we were in the process of turning a solemn and private moment into a farce with a cast of thousands.[22]

When JJ arrives with pizza they agree to take a 30-minute pause. After sharing their stories, they decide to delay the jumping for a while and see if they can help each other instead, starting with looking for Jess' boyfriend Chas. 'It wasn't much of a plan, really. But it was the only plan we had, so all we could do was try and make it work'.[23]

Forming an incongruous, shambolic but at least semi-competent self-help group, they survive a joint holiday in Tenerife and two reunions on the roof of Toppers' House. Step by step they keep on going. Maureen joins a quiz team and finds a job with a newsagent. JJ takes up busking. Martin begins a new career as a teacher. Jess starts a new relationship and makes peace with her parents. They all find ordinary yet serviceable new reasons to stay alive, at least for the time being.

In Matt Haig's *The Midnight Library*, Nora Seed decides at 22 minutes past 11 one rainy evening that her life is full of regrets, and no longer has any value at all: it is time for her to die. She takes an overdose. To her surprise she finds herself in a strange library with an infinite number of books, in the company of Mrs Elm, her former schoolteacher. Mrs Elm explains:

> 'Between life and death there is a library', she said. And within the library, the shelves go on for ever. Every book provides a chance to try another life you could have lived. To see how things would be different if you had made other choices. [...] Would you have done anything different if you had the chance to undo your regrets?'[24]

Haig builds his narrative on the basis of theories of multiverses, which comprise everything that exists, the entirety of space, time matter, energy and information. Within these parallel universes we each have an infinite range of choices. As we have lived a separate existence based on every possible choice we may have made, we have already experienced an infinite number of different lives. So Nora is able to try out multiple alternate lives, including Olympic swimmer, wife and mother, rock star, glaciologist, vineyard owner, dog walker and academic philosopher. Along the way she gradually loses her many regrets, her sense of guilt at how she has failed other people. A terrifying encounter with a polar bear helps her to realise she doesn't want to die: she wants to live, but to live differently.

She has the option to continue to live each of these alternate lives permanently. Some of them are very appealing, but she eventually decides to return to the one she started with. She wakes up at 1 minute and 27 seconds after midnight, vomits profusely, and 2 minutes later asks her neighbour to call an ambulance. She realises that regret is the problem, not life as she has lived it.

> 'It's not the lives we regret not living that are the real problem' she writes. 'It is the regret itself. It's the regret that makes us shrivel and wither and feel like our own and other people's worst enemy. [...] While we are alive we always contain a future of multifarious possibility'.[25]

I find myself using 'serious playfulness' a lot with patients in distress. One recent conversation about whether an older woman should dispose of her old sofa or herself at the local refuse collection centre led to a mutual fit of giggles; so, did a discussion about whether an anxious young man with a creaking neck would end up like Headless Humphrey in the TV series *Ghosts*. If we can find ways to laugh together at the ridiculous curveballs that life throws at us, it somehow offers us a little detachment, and the chance to look at things differently. And I sometimes wonder how Charlie would have responded to the multifarious possibilities available to her in her own midnight library. I like to imagine, from the book she had by her bedside when she died, that she would have loved to roam across Michael Moorcock's multiverse. Maybe she would have become a companion to the eternal champion, serving the cosmic balance in the eternal battle between law and chaos.[26] Or maybe she would have rewound her own story, finding fulfilment in her singing career, and choosing to be involved with someone who cherished rather than demeaned her.

I Can't Wrap This Up

Andrew Bennett explores the ways in which literature from the beginning of the twentieth century has responded to suicide as 'an increasingly normalized but incessantly baffling phenomenon'. His main concern is whether literary

reading may inform – and perhaps assist – those closely involved with
the lives and deaths of others. For many writers 'the generation or production
or exploitation of empathy […] is what the novel is *for*'. He proposes an
identificatory ethic of novelistic care, tracing back at least to George Eliot
(and I would add Tolstoy here), for whom paying attention outside of oneself
constituted 'the raw material of moral sentiment'. However, the impact of
such literary discourse is neither simple nor straightforward. Reading and
enhanced empathy do not necessarily, in Bennett's view, bring comfort
and relief:

> what is singular about literary novels is their tendency not only to
> encourage but also actively to confound empathy; it is not just that they
> complicate and refine such responses but that they may also resist,
> undermine and disrupt them.[27]

The contemporary novel 'can help us to grasp the limits of our
relationships – empathic, altruistic or otherwise – with those other people,
mired in or enmeshed with whose lives we cannot help but live and die'.[28]
But it cannot give us all the answers. We have seen already how Leopold
Bloom continues to wrestle with implications of his father's suicide 18 years
previously.

Although literature is the space in which everything can be said, yet
it also the space 'in which nothing can finally be justified or explained'.
Bennett asks himself, and us – and perhaps George Eliot and Tolstoy –
a series of highly charged questions. How does telling the story get the sight
of it out of your head? What do you gain? 'What is the benefit? What *good*
is done?'

These questions, which surface when we are faced with Tolstoy's graphic
description of the final moments of Anna Karenina's life, are strongly
relevant when we attempt to engage with the American novelist and literary
academic David Foster Wallace, whose spiralling sense of isolation, boredom
and the futility of existence plays itself out across the many pages of his two
major novels *Infinite Jest* and *The Pale King*. For Wallace the fundamentals of
existence, the intrinsic dullness of life, involve some 'deeper type of pain',
from which we need stimulation to distract ourselves. 'The key is the ability,
whether innate or conditioned, to find the other side of the rote, the picayune,
the meaningless, the repetitive, the pointlessly complex. To be, in a word,
unborable'.[29] Lots of bored people working for the internal revenue service
inhabit the pages of *The Pale King*, boringly trying to theorise boredom. After
many twists and turns, almost infinite digressions, and with the help of new
age eastern philosophy, in his notes on his unfinished novel Wallace attempts

to bring his characters, his readers and himself to a position of quasi-mystical transcendence through boredom to bliss:

> It turns out that bliss – a second-by-second joy' + gratitude at the gift of being alive, conscious – lies on the other side of crushing, crushing boredom. Pay close attention to the most tedious things you can find (tax returns, televised golf) and in waves, a boredom like you've never known will wash over you and just about kill you. Ride these out, and its like stepping from black and white into colour. Like water after days in the desert. Constant bliss in every atom.[30]

I recognise the sense of bliss that Wallace describes here. These moments are real, utterly real, but oh so fleeting. For me, there is floating down the tree-lined river near our French home, immersed in the rich solitude of nature; and standing with my son Michael at Intipunku (the gateway of the sun), looking down on the majesty of Machu Picchu. For Tolstoy's Levin, there is finding himself totally in tune with mowing the grass on his estate:

> The longer Levin mowed, the more often he felt those moment of oblivion during which it was no longer his arms that swung the scythe, but the scythe itself that lent motion to his whole body, full of life and conscious of itself and, as if by magic, without a thought of it, the work got rightly and neatly done on its own. These were the most blissful moments.[31]

And for Hopkins, as we have seen, there is his

>   dapple-dawn-drawn Falcon, in his riding
> Of the rolling level underneath him steady air, and striding
> High there, how he rung upon the rein of a wimpling wing
> In his ecstasy![32]

At last, we might reasonably conclude, Wallace has made his peace with life and the world. Resolution is achieved, meaning discovered. But before *The Pale King* was completed, at the age of 46, Wallace hanged himself at home, on his patio, to be discovered by his wife and his beloved dogs.

Perhaps he never quite achieved that state of blissful transcendence. Perhaps he did, but its ephemeral nature was too hard to bear. Perhaps, as his friend Jonathan Franzen observed, Wallace killed himself to prove he didn't deserve to be loved, committing a crime that was its own punishment.[33] Perhaps, as Andrew Bennett has suggested to me,[34] his failure to finish his novel – and even arguably his decision to end his own life – related to his sense that he was unable, with integrity, finally to get his characters or himself to this point of transcendence. Perhaps, perhaps, perhaps.... We will never know.

My next point of transformation is, therefore, a more cautious one. No matter how much our literary reading may enhance our sense of empathy, the suicide of another person with whom we have had a relationship – whether as family member, friend or patient – will always remain a 'traumatically intractable conundrum'. As Karen Green puts in her memoir of Wallace – her husband – 'I can't wrap this up'.[35]

We can neither tidy it away nor ever be finished with it. My patient Leigh talks to me about the incomprehensible suicide of her daughter Elle, now more than six years ago, in the midst of so much apparent joy in her life. She 'was overwhelmed with a sense of dread' when Elle's 15th birthday arrived. 'I didn't want her to turn fifteen. I knew I was going to lose her. My soul knew'. Elle had concerns about body dysmorphia, but there was nothing to suggest she found these intolerable. Guilt comes and goes in cycles, but Leigh knows it's not her fault. She was devastated, but not ashamed. 'You're not to blame' she says. But that is at best a partial consolation for her: it means 'you've no control over it happening again. You're constantly afraid it's going to happen to one of your other children'.

What Good Is Done?

There may yet be some consolation for us to find here, and at least a partial answer to Bennett's question 'What *good* is done?' If we can accept that it is impossible to fully understand why someone close to us has decided to kill themselves, it may be that – one day – literary reading enables us to find the grace to move beyond our guilt, our anger, our distress, to grant ourselves forgiveness for our ignorance and to carry on with the business of living our own lives.

Leigh finds no benefit from conventional religion, but has gained a lot from other spiritual sources. 'Religion has nothing to offer', she tells me, 'but there is more than this. Elle is still out there somewhere'. She had a wonderful singing voice, and Leigh connects with her through the lyrics of Rascal Flatts' *Why*:

Oh I had no clue you were masking a troubled soul.
God only knows what went wrong,
and why you'd leave the stage in the middle of a song.[36]

She reads voraciously, usually stories from others similarly bereaved. She has been most influenced by Annie Kagan's *The Afterlife of Billy Fingers*, with its tale of Annie's 'good for nothing' brother, who contacts her early one morning, a few weeks after his death in a traffic accident, to tell her he's drifting through the universe with a loving, beneficent divine presence twinkling all around him.[37] Leigh believes we all have 'soul contracts': we come down here on earth with a set of goals. 'Our experience is predetermined'.

Who knows, we may even flourish, like Jane Fairchild in Graham Swift's *Mothering Sunday*,[38] and the playwright in Maggie O'Farrell's *Hamnet*.[39]

The narrative of *Mothering Sunday* centres around and spirals out from the day of the title, in March 1924. Jane, a foundling orphan placed in domestic service, is in a secret relationship with Paul Sheringham, the youngest son of a wealthy neighbouring family. A fortnight hence Paul is to be married, move to London and become a lawyer. Today is the last time they will ever be together 'in the supreme region of utter mutual nakedness'. Jane is getting ready to lose Paul, as he dresses in his 'going away clothes', driving off to an arranged lunch in a nearby hotel with his and his fiancée's families. But he never arrives. Leaving it late and in a hurry, he takes shortcut on a minor road and drives straight into an oak tree on the apex of a right-hand bend.

A tragic accident is what the inquest finds, and what the families wished to believe. But it was a day of bright sunshine. Paul knew the road well, there was no evidence of motor malfunction or stray animals. Perhaps he could not face the future mapped out for him, and chose a different ending.

Either way, it is a crossroads in Jane's own life:

> [...] one very warm day in March when she was twenty-two and she had wandered around a house without a shred on – naked, you might say, as on the day she was born – and had felt both more herself, more Jane Fairchild than she'd ever felt before, yet also, as never before, like some visiting ghost. Had felt, you might say, what it truly means to be put down in this world, placed so to speak, on its extraordinary doorstep.[40]

It is the day she becomes a writer. When told of Paul's death she, as a servant, has no right to express her grief in public. 'Her face had momentarily flooded, before she drenched it anyway with cold water. She might even have stifled a scream'. She finds solace in the novels of Joseph Conrad, another secret agent adept at slipping between worlds. Her life moves on, to Oxford, to marriage (for a while), and to writing: writing with an awareness of the inconstancy of language – 'words are only words, just bits of air' – and with the realisation, crystallised on that warm day in March, that 'many things in life – oh so many more than we think – can never be explained at all'.

In *Hamnet*, we find the narrative circling around the death of Shakespeare's son at the age of 11. O'Farrell portrays this historical event it as the result of a deliberate, conscious choice on Hamnet's part: to give up his own life in order to save the life of his identical twin sister Judith, who is gravely ill with the plague and all but given up for dead by her family. For many years the two of them have played games involving swapping roles, so that even their parents and close are not sure who is who. Hamnet extrapolates this game to its ultimate, utterly serious conclusion: 'It will be easy for Death to make a mistake, to take him in her place'. He lies next to her on her straw pallet.

> He breathes in. He breathes out. He turns his head and breathes into the whorls of her ear; he breathes in his strength, his health, his all. You will stay is what he whispers, and I will go. He sends these words into her. I want you to take my life. It shall be yours, I give it to you.
>
> They cannot both be live: he sees this and she sees this. There is not enough life, enough air, enough blood for both of them. Perhaps there never was. And if either of them is to live, it must be her. He wills it. He grips the sheet, tight, in both hands. He, Hamnet, decrees it. It shall be.[41]

This act of Hamnet's is the epitome of Durkheim's altruistic suicide, sacrificing his life for the sake of another member of his social group.[42] Yet it is both inexplicable and devastating for his whole family. His mother Agnes, like the widow in Williams' lament, all but gives up the will to live in her desire to be reunited with him. His father returns to his theatrical work in London, and for years can write nothing but comedies and historical plays. Tragedy is too overwhelming to be borne. Their relationship deteriorates.

But then, some five years later, Agnes learns indirectly of her husband's new play, entitled *Hamlet*. Shocked and fascinated by this news, she travels to London to watch the first performance. There she sees her husband playing the ghost of the dead king, and to her utter astonishment, her son brought back to 'life' on the stage:

> It is him. It is not him. It is him. It is not him. The thought swings like a hammer through her. Her son, her Hamnet or Hamlet, is dead, buried in the churchyard. He died while he was still a child. He is now only white, stripped bones in a grave. Yet this is him, grown into a near man, as he would be now, had he lived, on the stage, walking with her son's gait. Talking in her son's voice, speaking words written for him by her son's father.[43]

In O'Farrell's telling, Shakespeare has channelled his sorrow, resurrecting their son's life through this sublime example of dramatic intensity. Writing, the act of artistic creation, now becomes not only a source of solace, a means of coming to terms with the grief of inexplicable loss, but also – and so much more – the opportunity to find new meanings, fresh inspiration: for the author, for those (like Agnes) who love him, for that first audience at the Globe and, eventually, for all of us.

Leigh is flourishing too, in her own way. She is pursuing a successful international teaching career. Her surviving son is off to university later this year. She has a new relationship and twin baby boys: 'Elle's soul is in them now'. In Elle's honour she has set up the Mirror of Hope Foundation. Its mission is to highlight and reduce the suffering caused by self-harming and body dysmorphic disorders. It also exists to provide help and support to people of any age who are finding life hard to navigate, regardless of how that manifests.[44]

And Then We Shall Dwell Together

My final transformation concerns how support from others, when we are confronting the dilemma of our own existence, can make the difference between life and death for us.

We have already seen this dynamic in operation, in the relationships between Kitty and Varenka in *Anna Karenina*, between Nora and her teacher/librarian in *The Midnight Library*, and between the motley crew who find themselves together on New Year's Eve on Toppers Tower in *A Long Way Down*: all accidental relationships, developing amongst people coming together by chance. We can also gain immense, life-saving support closer to home. To illustrate this, I present two stories from long ago, the first from the Norse sagas and the second from ancient Egypt.

Egil Skallagrimsson, was a tenth-century Viking Age sorcerer, berserker and farmer – and an exceptionally skilled poet. On one occasion, he saved his own life by composing a poem in praise of king Erik Bloodaxe, while imprisoned by Erik's men in Northumbria, on the very night before he was due to be beheaded. The poem, called Höfuðlausn or Head-Ransom, was so good that the king spared Egil's life.

Sonatorrek, on the other hand, is the poem that Egil's daughter Torgedur tricks him into composing when he has decided to end his life out of despair after having lost two of his sons.[45] Torgerdur saves his life by luring him into one of his favourite activities, writing poetry, as a way of both re-engaging with the world and re-establishing his sense of meaning.

After the death of his son Bodvar, the grieving Egil takes to his bed and refuses to eat or drink. Torgedur is summoned by her mother to help. When she arrives at her father's home she announces in a loud voice;

> I have had no evening meal, nor will I do so until I go to join Freyja. I know no better course of action than my father's. I do not want to live after my father and brother are dead.

She lies down in the bed next to her father, and Egil is pleased with the compassion she displays. She persuades him to try some edible seaweed, telling him that it is bad for him and will hasten his demise. Then she tricks him into drinking milk, telling him that it was water that she called for. After convincing him that they have both been tricked, she pushes her father a stage further:

> What will we do now? Our plan has failed. Now I want us to stay alive, father, long enough for you to compose a poem in Bodvar's memory and I will carve it on a rune-stick. Then we can die if we want to. I doubt whether your son Thorstein would ever compose a poem for Bodvar, and it is unseemly if his memory is not honoured, because I do not expect us to be sitting there at the feast when it is.[46]

Egil agrees, and composes the poem *Sonatorrek* (the irreparable loss of sons) in honour of his dead son:

> My boy was borne off
> By a burning sea-fever,
> The searing storm
> Was his sea-sickness:
> My son, who shunned
> All spite and slander -
> I must weep.
> [...]
>
> The end is all.
> Even now
> High on the headland
> Hel stands and waits,
> Life fades, and I must fall
> And face my own end
> Not in misery and mourning
> But with a man's heart.[47]

The combination of care from his daughter and engagement in the imaginative process of writing this poem enables Egil to recover from his grief. He rises from his bed and showers Tordegur with presents as she departs.

Sometime between 1937 and 1759 BCE, during the Twelfth Dynasty of the Middle Kingdom of ancient Egypt, a papyrus was created which is currently the earliest surviving literary document about suicide. It depicts the dialogue between a man and his soul, or Ba. Ba was that essence of the human which retained the ability to move freely in the afterlife between the world of gods and the corpse. It enabled the reanimation of the man's living existence after the death of the physical body.

The papyrus was bought in 1843 by archaeologist Karl Lepsius, and can now be found in a museum in Berlin. It comprises 155 vertical columns of hieroglyphs. The first portion is missing and there are lots of gaps, hence there have been a number of different interpretation and translations. Here I follow the translation adopted by Miriam Lichtheim, and present quotations taken from her panoramic study of ancient Egyptian literature.[48]

The man explains that he is tired of living. His reputation has been trashed:

> Lo, my name reeks – more than carrion smell on summer days of burning sky. Lo, my name reeks – more than a catch of fish on fishing days of burning sky. Lo, my name reeks, more than that of a wife about whom lies are told to the husband.

His belongingness is severely thwarted. He is all alone, deserted by past friends in an evil, uncaring world:

> To whom shall I speak today? Brothers are mean. The friends of today do not love. To whom shall I speak today? I am burdened with grief for lack of an intimate. To whom shall I speak today? Wrong roams the earth and ends not.

He decided to end his life by going to 'the West', the place of death, and find release from his suffering. Death will bring welcome relief:

> Death is in my sight today, like the recovery of a sick man, like going out into the open after a confinement. Death is in my sight today, like the odour of myrrh, like sitting under an awning on a breezy day. Death is in my sight today, like the passing away of rain, like the return of men to their houses from an expedition.

In death he will also find revenge against his enemies, enjoy wealth beyond measure, and then receive the wisdom of the gods:

> Truly, he who is yonder will be a living god, punishing the evildoer's crime. Truly, he who is yonder will stand in the sun-bark, making its bounty flow to the temples. Truly, he who is yonder will be a wise man, not barred from appealing to Re when he speaks.

Ba is unimpressed by the man's talk of suicide. He is convinced it will lead him to total annihilation instead of resurrection and immortal bliss. He engages in an earnest debate with the man about the wisdom and inevitability of his proposed actions. He dismisses the man's assurance that proper burial arrangements make everything alright, declaring that death is a sad business and fine tombs are of no benefit. He encourages the man to take up a life of pleasure – 'Follow the feast day, forget worry' – and tells him stories designed to illustrate the danger of embarking on such a course of action before its due time. In the first story, a man loses wife and children to crocodiles: but the man mourns for his dead children more than wife because their lives were too short: 'I grieve for my children broken in the egg, who have seen the face of the crocodile before they have lived'. In the second, very brief tale, a man demands dinner before his wife has prepared it: the moral being that impatience, wanting death before it is time, is irrational.

Eventually, Ba persuades the man to set worries aside, and carry on living until it is his appointed time to die. Then he will be able to keep the man company into the next life:

> Now, throw complaint in the wood pile, you my comrade, my brother! Whether you offer on the brazier, whether you bear down on life, as you say, love me here when you have set aside the West! But when it is wished that you attain the West, that your body joins the earth, I shall alight after you have become weary, and then we shall dwell together.

The psychiatrist Chris Thomas considers this text to be the first suicide note in history, He sees it as the writing of a 'severely psychotically depressed man with feelings of persecution and self-depreciation who also undoubtedly shows strong suicidal tendencies'.[49] Although he is right to draw attention to the man's profound pessimism and world-weariness, I think Thomas' interpretation of the text as a whole is flawed. For me, this dialogue distils the essence of what I wish to demonstrate in this chapter, and indeed in the book as a whole. It confronts the dilemma of existence in the face of grief and loss, and crucially offers us a point of transformation: one based on intimate relationship.

The lyrical form of repeated phrases (Lo my name reeks [...] To whom shall I speak today [...] Death is in my sight today [...] Truly, he who is yonder [...]), linked with a series of evocative metaphors, creates a series of powerful images which deeply engage the reader or the listener with the man's profound distress, his sense of alienation from the world and himself.

And then, through the device of poetic dialogue, we are shown a means of recovery, and the re-emergence of a sense of agency.[50] Life may well be the occasion of many sorrows, but it is a limited and treasured resource, to be enjoyed while we can.

Relief from suffering is possible, in Yordan Chobanov's interpretation of the text, 'through confession, sharing that which is troubling the person with a man of pure heart'.[51] While this phrasing is uncomfortably gendered, it does have resonance with the *anamchara* (soul friend) of the Celtic wisdom traditions[52]: a compassionate presence with the ability to read a person's heart, and a willingness to accompany them into the depths of darkness, exploring the landscape there together.

It also inspires me in my reflections on the therapeutic potential of the encounters between doctor and patient, and provides an important final piece of evidence in support of this social point of transformation. I often find myself, in conversation with a person who is tired of life, taking a role not entirely dissimilar to that of the Ba: acknowledging their pain and suffering, suggesting reasons to stay alive and – above all – staying close by them as they explore new ways of being.

The term 'holding' has been proposed by Simon Cocksedge for those doctor–patient relationships which involve establishing and maintaining a trusting, constant and reliable relationship that is concerned with ongoing support without expectation of cure.[53] This is an essential and under-recognised element of the health professional's work that deserves to be named and valued. Indeed, for several patients in the depths of despair, I have made the offer to 'hold on to your hope for you' until they feel able to reclaim it for themselves. In that moment, I am perhaps close to becoming their Ba.

Points of Transformation

In this chapter, I have shown how self-destruction is not our only option when faced with despair. Literary texts and poetry offer us points of transformation, opportunities to think and act differently.

With Al Alvarez we may acknowledge that, while suicide may be an everyday temptation, it offers no resolution or salvation, and is (most likely) merely the end of experience. We may be persuaded by Stevie Smith that death is to be earned, not grasped before its time; and find resolve in the ways in which she, along with Zbigniew Herbert and Seamus Heaney, confront the seriousness of living through personally and politically troubled times. We may come to realise, with Jane Fairchild and Hamnet's parents, that it is possible not only to survive but even to flourish despite the inexplicable death of someone we have loved; and with Nora Seed, that life has infinite possibilities. We may find help from more or less expected sources, whether from a modern, earth-bound, therapeutic version of Ba, a wise and tricky daughter like Torgerdur, or other people contemplating death on top of a high-rise building.

The poetic and literary texts I have chosen to focus on here are simply those which have resonance for me. They provide me with a set of ideas and inspirations with which to confront the dilemma of existence, starting points for new conversations with patients, loved ones and sometimes even myself. I am fully aware of and entirely unapologetic for the eclectic nature of my selection. I am with at one with Matt Haig here, in his 33rd piece of advice on how to live:

> Read Emily Dickinson. Read Grahame Greene. Read Italo Calvino. Read Maya Angelou. Read anything you want. Just read. Books are possibilities. They are escape routes. They give you options when you have none. Each one can be a home for an uprooted mind.[54]

My hope is that this chapter, and indeed this book as a whole, will encourage you to reflect on your own reading. I would love to hear from you about how your literary reading has been transformative for your own experiences of grief, loss and despair. Perhaps we can, together, create an ever-expanding set of therapeutic literary resources.

Notes

1 William Carols Williams, 'The Widows Lament in Springtime'. *Sour Grapes* (Boston: Four Seas Publication, 1921), 43.
2 James Joyce, *Selected Letters*, ed. Richard Ellman (Ithaca, NY: Cornell University Press, 1989), 73–75.
3 James Joyce, *Dubliners* (Harmondsworth: Penguin Modern Classics, 1972), 216, 220.
4 James Joyce, *Ulysses* (Harmondsworth: Penguin Modern Classics, 1960), 98–99.
5 Joyce, Ulysses, ibid., 499.
6 Andrew Bennett, *Suicide Century: Literature and Suicide from James Joyce to David Foster Wallace* (Cambridge: Cambridge University Press, 2017), 106.
7 Alfred Alvarez, *The Savage God: A Study of Suicide* (New York: Bantam Edition, Random House, 1973).
8 Wilfrid Owen, *Collected Letters* (Oxford: Oxford University Press, 1967), 521.

9 Alvarez, *Savage God*, ibid., 268, 270.
10 Stevie Smith, *Novel on Yellow Paper* (London: Jonathan Cape, 1936), 159.
11 Dead Poets Live. Accessed 10 March 2021. https://www.shakespearesglobe.com/whats-on/dead-poets-live-2021/.
12 Bennett, *Suicide Century*, ibid., 128.
13 Stevie Smith, *Collected Poems and Drawings of Stevie Smith*, ed. William May (London: Faber, 2015), 207.
14 William Wootten, *The Alvarez Generation* (Liverpool: Liverpool University Press, 2015).
15 Alfred Alvarez, *Where Did It All Go Right?* (London: Richard Cohen Books, 1999), 209–210.
16 Peter Porter, 'Poetry and Madness', in *Saving from the Wreck* (Nottingham: Trent Books, 2001), 2.
17 Peter Porter, *Collected Poems 1,1961–1981* (Oxford, Oxford University Press 1999), 338.
18 Pam Ayres, 'They Should Have Asked my Husband'. Accessed 16 July 2021. https://pamayres.com/poems/.
19 Wisława Szymborska, *Map: Collected and Last Poems* (New York: Houghton Mifflin Harcourt, 2016).
20 Zbigniew Herbert, 'Damastes (Also Known as Procrustes) Speaks', *Selected Poems*, trans John and Bogdana Carpenter (Oxford: Oxford University Press, 1974), 48.
21 Iona Heath, 'Subjectivity of patients and doctors', in *Person-Centred Primary Care*, ed. Christopher Dowrick (Abingdon: Routledge, 2018), 80.
22 Nick Hornby, *A Long Way Down* (London: Penguin Books, 2006), 19.
23 Hornby, *Long Way Down*, ibid., 42.
24 Matt Haig, *The Midnight Library* (London: Canongate, 2020), 29.
25 Haig, *Midnight Library*, ibid., 277–78.
26 Michael Moorcock, *The Sundered Worlds* (Radford: Wilder Publications, 2011).
27 Bennett, *Suicide Century*, ibid., 57.
28 Bennett, *Suicide Century*, ibid., 164.
29 David Foster Wallace, *The Pale King: An Unfinished Novel* (New York: Little Brown and Company, 2011), 437–38.
30 Wallace, *The Pale King*, ibid., 546.
31 Leo Tolstoy, *Anna Karenina*, trans. Richard Pevear and Larissa Volokhonsky (London: Penguin Books 2003), 252.
32 Gerard Manley Hopkins, 'The Windhover' *Poems and Prose of Gerard Manley Hopkins*, ed. William Gardner (London: Penguin Books, 1968), 30.
33 Jonathan Franzen, 'Farther Away: *Robinson Crusoe*, David Foster Wallace, and the Island of Solitude', *New Yorker*. April 18, 2011.
34 Andrew Bennett, personal communication, 2 April 2021.
35 Karen Green, *Bough Down* (Los Angeles: Siglio, 2013), 184.
36 Rascal Flatts: 'Why'. Accessed 24 July 2021. https://open.spotify.com/album/6xDwYyGCOkD2t9GuBikEL8?ighlight=spotify:track:5aFQ8js9G12JzIJN9Ct9ET.
37 Annie Kagan, *The Afterlife of Billy Fingers* (London: Hodder & Stoughton, 2014).
38 Graham Swift, *Mothering Sunday* (London: Simon & Schuster, 2016).
39 Maggie O'Farrell, *Hamnet* (London: Tinder Press, 2020).
40 Swift, Mothering Sunday, ibid., 98–99.
41 O'Farrell, *Hamnet*, ibid., 201.
42 Emile Durkheim, *Suicide: A Study in Sociology*, trans. John Spaulding and George Simpson (London: Routledge, 2005).

43 O'Farrell, *Hamnet*, ibid., 364–65.

44 Mirror of Hope. Accessed 24 July 2021. https://www.facebook.com/mirrorofhope1999.

45 I am grateful to Stefan Hjørleifsson for drawing this story to my attention.

46 Snorri Sturluson, 'Egil's Saga', in *The Sagas of the Icelanders*, ed. Örnólfur Thorsson, trans. Bernard Scudder (New York: Penguin Books, 2001), 151–52.

47 Snorri Sturluson, *Egil's Saga*, Penguin Classics version trans. Hermann Pálsson and Paul Edwards (London: Penguin Books, 1976).

48 Miriam Lichtheim, *Ancient Egyptian Literature, Volume 1: The Old and Middle Kingdoms* (Oakland: University of California Press, 2006), 164–69.

49 Chris Thomas, 'First suicide note?' *British Medical Journal* 281 (1980): 284–85.

50 Richard Parkinson, *Poetry and Culture in Middle Kingdom Egypt* (London: Equinox, 2002).

51 Yordan Chobanov, 'A New Interpretation of the Dialog of a Man and His Ba'. *Journal of Egyptological Studies* 4 (2015): 84–97.

52 John O'Donohue, *Anam Cara: A Book of Celtic Wisdom* (New York: Cliff Street Books, 1997).

53 Simon Cocksedge et al., 'Holding Relationships in Primary Care: A Qualitative Exploration of Doctors' and Patients' Perceptions'. *British Journal of General Practice* 61, no. 589 (2011): e484–91.

54 Matt Haig, *Reasons to Stay Alive* (London: Canongate, 2015), 242.

Chapter 6

CREATING *RAISONS D'ETRE*

To be, or not to be: that is the question:
Whether 'tis nobler in the mind to suffer
The slings and arrows of outrageous fortune,
Or to take arms against a sea of troubles,
And by opposing end them? To die: to sleep;
No more; and by a sleep to say we end
The heart-ache and the thousand natural shocks
That flesh is heir to, 'tis a consummation
Devoutly to be wish'd. To die, to sleep;
To sleep: perchance to dream: ay, there's the rub;
For in that sleep of death what dreams may come
When we have shuffled off this mortal coil,
Must give us pause: there's the respect
That makes calamity of so long life.

For who would bear the whips and scorns of time,
The oppressor's wrong, the proud man's contumely,
The pangs of despised love, the law's delay,
The insolence of office and the spurns
That patient merit of the unworthy takes,
When he himself might his quietus make
With a bare bodkin? Who would fardels bear,
To grunt and sweat under a weary life,
But that the dread of something after death,
The undiscover'd country from whose bourn
No traveller returns, puzzles the will
And makes us rather bear those ills we have
Than fly to others that we know not of?

Thus conscience does make cowards of us all;
And thus the native hue of resolution

Is sicklied o'er with the pale cast of thought,
And enterprises of great pith and moment
With this regard their currents turn awry,
And lose the name of action.

A Vain, Fruitless, and Self-Contradictory Effort

In this famous soliloquy from Act 3 Scene 1, Shakespeare's Hamlet clearly didn't think his existence amounted to anything worthwhile, bombarded as it was with the slings and arrows of outrageous fortune, with heartache and a thousand natural shocks, with the whips and scorns of time, with the oppressor's wrong and the pangs of disprized love. Why should he continue with the grunt and sweat of his weary life?

We have seen this question raised many times before in this book, whether in the lamentations of the Man to his Ba, in the terminal boredom of David Foster Wallace, in the existential distress of Anna Karenina and Constantin Levin or in the spiritual weariness of Gerard Manley Hopkins. And we find it expressed in philosophical terms, most notably by the nineteenth century's prince of pessimism, Arthur Schopenhauer.

For Schopenhauer, there is 'only one inborn error', the idea that 'we exist in order to be happy'. Dying is 'the real aim of life'. 'At the moment of dying everything is decided which through the whole course of life was only prepared and introduced'. Everything we have strived for, the effort of living, 'has been a vain, fruitless, and self-contradictory effort, to have returned from which is a deliverance'.[1] The tragedy of being human is that through reflection both our happiness and our misery are exaggerated. We are subject to 'momentary and sometimes even fatal ecstasy' and also to the 'the depths of suicide and despair'.[2] Thinking in itself is thus, originally, suicidal.

Adulthood occurs when you realise you may not be leading a charmed life.

> In early youth we sit before the impending course of our life like children at the theatre before the curtain is raised, who sit there in happy and excited expectations of the things that are to come. It is a blessing that we do not know what will actually come. For to the man who knows, the children may at times appear to be like innocent delinquents who are condemned not to death, it is true, but to life and have not yet grasped the purport of their sentence.[3]

And we find Søren Kierkegaard, Schopenhauer's Danish contemporary, proposing that despair is 'man's advantage over the beast [...] for it bespeaks the infinite erectness or loftiness of his being spirit'.[4] Despair may take many forms: being unaware that we have an authentic self; believing that we do have a self but that it is somehow unworthy and wishing for to be different; despair in the possibility of comfort from God (as we saw so vividly expressed in the Hopkins' *No Worse* and *I Wake and Feel*); and the final level (which Hopkins' eventually resists in *Carrion Comfort*) of revelling in our despair, of believing that our own pain somehow elevates us above the common mass of humanity. Kierkegaard believed this final level was most often to be found in poets: we have seen in the previous chapter how it was expressed in the writings of Sylvia Plath, Stevie Smith and Al Alvarez; yet strongly countered by Peter Porter.

These arguments have been extended more recently by the South African philosopher David Benatar who proposes – with deliberate provocation – that it would be better for us never to have been born because of the harms necessarily associated with human existence. Existence always holds harm, even if it is merely the slightest of painful pinpricks. Non-existence is preferable because it entails no harm, along with no experience of the absence of any benefits that existence might offer.[5] And we can take this proposition a stage further by considering not only the individual but also the global benefits of human non-existence, given the environmental havoc we are collectively wreaking on our planet.

So why, actually, should we bother to stay alive? In this chapter, I will consider how literary reflections on the dilemma of existence may be complemented by philosophical approaches in creating reasons to be.

The only reason Hamlet can find to be rather than not to be is his dread of something worse after death. That undiscovered country puzzles his will. He would rather bear the ills he has than deliberately choose to fly to others that he knows not of. Shakespeare is deliberately and reasonably opaque about the form and content of the undiscovered country from whose bourn no traveller returns. For his audiences, who believed suicide to be a mortal sin, the prospects of eternal damnation in the fires of hell were far from appealing. For those of his contemporaries familiar with renaissance literature and the poetic vision of Dante, where suicides found themselves in the seventh circle of the inferno, transformed into gnarled, condemned and cursed trees to be perpetually tormented by Harpies, Hamlet's argument may well have had considerable merit. But it is the most negative possible justification for staying alive.

We have already seen, in previous chapters, how the literary imagination offers us other reasons for making the choice to live when faced with the dilemma of existence. Even if the consequence of death is merely oblivion, we may agree with Al Alvarez that suicide is nothing more than the denial of experience and provides no solutions. We may come to share Stevie Smith's view that death is not to be snatched prematurely, but earned through the endurance of a worthwhile life. We may find strength through the poetry of Gerard Manley Hopkins to not choose not to be and leave root-room for self-compassion. Or we may follow Tolstoy and Levin in looking beyond ourselves and seek to do good in the world.

Philosophical inquiry can support and extend these perspectives. Stevie Smith's view, as expressed in *Study to Deserve Death*, is close to the philosophical term known as deontology, which asserts that we have a duty or obligation to do the right thing – in this case to stay alive – regardless of its consequences. We can counter David Benatar's anti-natalism with the argument that future children may be better off experiencing the harms and benefits of life rather than never having the opportunity to experience anything,[6] or to ameliorate the world in which they find themselves.

Schopenhauer, perhaps surprisingly, was not in favour of suicide as a response to the misery of human existence. He believed we all have a fundamental will to life. He accepted that thought of suicide is a fundamental feature of human existence, but because it involves destruction of the body, the phenomenon of the will to life, people are usually deterred. The suicide wills life, but not *this* life. When a person destroys their existence as an individual, they are not by any means destroying their will to live. On the contrary, they would like to live if they could do so with satisfaction, if they could assert their will against the power of circumstance, but circumstances are sometimes too strong.[7] It is no coincidence that this is very much the position that Anna Karenina found herself in, caught between her unresolvable needs for her lover and her son, since Tolstoy was (at that period in his life) in turns fascinated and repulsed by Schopenhauer's views on the blind will to life, in opposition to a representation of the world produced by intelligence.[8]

Schopenhauer understood the world to be a thing in itself, a general universal Will, existing outside the subjective forms of space and time. Suffering is essential to all life, so the 'arbitrary destruction of an individual phenomenon' is futile and foolish because the thing in itself, the general universal Will, remains unaffected by the act, like a rainbow that remains 'unmoved, however rapidly the drops may change which sustain it for the moment'.[9] The individual act of suicide is an epiphenomenon, nothing more than 'the foam on the surface of human existence'.[10]

He does, however, offer us consolation in our miserable existence through the realisation that individuality is merely an illusion. The saint or great soul, in their ascetic practice, 'recognizes the whole, comprehends its essence, and finds that it is constantly passing away, caught up in vain strivings, inner conflict, and perpetual suffering'.[11] We can liberate ourselves from striving and suffering through recognition that the world in itself, free from the forms of space and time, is one.

Schopenhauer was notoriously bad-tempered in his dealings with fellow philosophers; nevertheless, he was one of the first Western philosophers to argue that compassion should be the basis of morality.[12] The fact that the world is such a miserable place should lead us to have sympathy for each other, as we are all in a similar plight:

> The conviction that the world, and therefore man too, is something which really ought not to exist is in fact calculated to instil in us indulgence towards one another: for what can be expected of beings placed in such a situation as we are? [This ...] reminds us of what are the most necessary of all things: tolerance, patience, forbearance and charity, which each of us needs and which each of us therefore owes.[13]

Kierkegaard was sceptical of Schopenhauer's motives in proposing an ethical approach to life which he did not himself adopt: he noted in his journals that Schopenhauer 'makes ethics into genius and although he prides himself quite enough on being a genius, it has not pleased him, or nature has not allowed him, to become a genius where asceticism and mortification are concerned'.[14] However, he did agree that an ethical existence, in which the individual becomes aware of and personally responsible for good and evil and of the need to form a commitment to oneself and others, is of greater value as a counter to despair than a purely aesthetic approach, whereby we pass through our lives in a largely unreflective way. He took this position a stage further by assuming religion, understood as the impulse towards an awareness of a transcendent power in the universe, to be the highest form of human existence. For Kierkegaard, as for Tolstoy and Hopkins, this involved commitment to and relationship with the Christian God.[15]

Schopenhauer was impressed the insights of Eastern thought, and had a statue of Buddha in his study. So it is no coincidence that his view is close to that of Buddhist philosophy, in particular to its first noble truth of *dukkha*:

> The noble truth of dukkha is this: birth is dukkha; ageing is dukkha; sickness is dukkha; death is dukkha; sorrow and lamentation, pain, grief and despair are dukkha; association with the unpleasant is dukkha; dissociation from the pleasant is dukkha; not to get what one wants is dukkha – in brief, the five aggregates of attachment are dukkha.[16]

The most popular English translation of dukkha is the word 'suffering', although this does not do justice to the depth and complexity of the concept.

In reality, there is no adequate English equivalent. In addition to suffering, dukkha has been variously translated as sorrow, frustration, unhappiness, anguish, stressfulness or unsatisfactoriness. It has also been translated as illness or dis-ease. Yet, it means a great deal more than any of these words. It refers not just to a specific state of mind but to the fundamental experience of human existence as characterised by transience, and all that arises from the experience of transience: an awareness of the impermanent and ephemeral nature of things, the temporality and finitude of life. Even happiness can be considered to be an aspect of dukkha, insofar as it is a transitory experience, based on attachments or achievements that themselves are also temporary.[17]

But this is not to assume that Buddhists have a pessimistic worldview.[18] Like Schopenhauer, their aspiration is to a view that is beyond either pessimism or optimism. They lead us in directions that transcend the sorts of experiences that cause us to question the value of our existence. Attachment to the self is a kind of dysfunction, and losing that attachment is liberation. No-self (*anattā*), the awareness that there is no permanent underlying substance that can be called a soul, is intimately connected to concern for the suffering of others.[19]

The Buddhist practice of *metta bhavana*, or compassion meditation, is a set of techniques designed to increase our interest in the happiness of others and our wish to relieve others' suffering. It begins with learning how to regulate our own thoughts and emotions and, like Gerard Manley Hopkins, find ways to develop compassion for ourselves.[20] It links with mid-twentieth-century Christian theology of relationships as the key to our distinctiveness as human beings: whether in the form of Karl Barth's 'being in encounter',[21] or the 'I:Thou' relationship of Martin Buber, the mutual holistic exchange of two beings (two lovers, an observer and a cat, the writer and a tree, or two strangers on a train) who meet without qualification or objectification of the other, and in the process finding that their own selves appear and grow as each recognises the other.[22] And in the sphere of the clinical consultation, it brings us to Ron Epstein's concept of 'shared mind', of the ways in which new ideas and perspectives, new hope of fresh possibilities, can emerge through sharing thoughts, feelings, perceptions, meanings and intentions among two or more people.[23]

Intentional Entity

I have previously proposed a concept of the self, deriving from two interacting components of coherence and engagement. I have argued that such an understanding of the self provides us with a basis for purposeful existence in the face of depression,[24,25] chronic ill-health and reduced mental capacity.[26] Reviewing these arguments in the context of suicide, and with the benefit of insights gained from my encounters with Tolstoy and Hopkins, I will now consider how our sense of coherence, our desire to persevere in our own being, is of fundamental importance but may at times become overwhelmed. I will suggest that engagement – whether communal, political or spiritual – may be the critical element in the existential preservation of the self, enabling us to rediscover or create reasons to be.

I start with an understanding of ourselves as coherent beings, neither wholly individualised on the one hand, nor illusory, fragmented or role-playing on the other hand. I assume that human life has a sense of unity throughout its whole extent, that we are fundamentally real and intrinsically valuable beings with the capacity to change and progress. I also propose that we have inherent agency, the capacity to lead our own lives, the power to make our own choices and decisions, to take intentional action in a given environment.[27]

I agree with Tim Bayne that to understand what it is like for me to be me, it is helpful to consider myself as an *intentional entity*, with streams of consciousness constructed around a single intentional object. He gives the example of himself sitting in a Cuban café in Paris:

> I have auditory experiences of various kinds: I can hear the bartender making a mojito; I can hear the dog behind me chasing his tail; and there's a rumba song playing somewhere on a stereo. I am enjoying visual experiences of various kinds: I can see these words as they appear in my notebook; I can see the notebook itself; and I have a blurry visual impression of those parts of the room that lie behind the notebook. Co-mingled with these auditory and visual experiences are olfactory experiences of various kinds (I can smell something roasting in the kitchen); bodily sensations of various kinds (I am aware of my legs under the chair; I can feel my fingers on the table); and a range of cognitive and affective experiences. The bartender is talking to an old woman at the bar, and I have a vague sense of understanding what he's saying. I am soon to embark on a lengthy trip, and a sense of anticipation colours my experiential state. Finally, I am enjoying conscious thoughts. I realise that the bar is about to close, and that I will be asked to leave if I stay for much longer.[28]

For Bayne, my self is a virtual centre of 'phenomenal gravity', 'an object whose identity is given by the intentional structure of the phenomenal field'. I appropriate to myself those experiences I am aware of. I assume that the character at the centre of my current stream of consciousness is the same as the character I am in contact with through my autobiographical memory.

In making that assumption we are 'not merely *tracking* ourselves but *creating* them'.[29] Like Jane Fairchild in *Mothering Sunday*, we are the creators of our own narratives, our own stories.

Desire Is the Very Essence of Man

I suggest that our sense of coherence is based on four elements: memory, imagination, curiosity and – above all – desire.

Memory is the principal means by which we demonstrate our sense of continuity to ourselves, linking thoughts and emotions in a way that produces a sense of self-coherence.[30] Memory can be traumatic, as in the case studies of Sigmund Freud where adverse childhood experiences return, in various guises, to haunt and control the lives and thoughts of his patients; or in our final encounter with Tolstoy's Vronsky, who cannot escape from the image of Anna's blood-covered body. But we can also turn memory into a source of energy. In the opening chapter of *Swann's Way*, Marcel Proust's narrator is feeling particular cold and miserable one day. His mother persuades him to soak a madeleine, a small cake in his cup of tea.

> No sooner had the warm liquid mixed with the crumbs touched my palate than a shiver ran through me and I stopped, intent upon the extraordinary thing that was happening to me. An exquisite pleasure had invaded my senses, something isolated, detached, with no suggestion of its origin. And at once the vicissitudes of life had become indifferent to me, its disasters innocuous, its brevity illusory – this new sensation having had the effect, which love has, of filling me with a precious essence; or rather this essence was not in me, it *was* me. I had ceased now to feel mediocre, contingent, mortal.

The sight of the madeleine crumbled into his tea was not in itself significant. Rather it was the direct sensations of smell and taste which, like souls outlasting the ruin of the body, elicit the sensation of joy and bring him into touch with the immense edifice of memories of the past, a past that had hitherto seemed completely lost to him, in this case a memory of himself as a child visiting his aunt on a Sunday morning. Once activated, memory blossoms. Like those Japanese paper shapes that come to life when placed in water, so his whole childhood, with all its sights and places and people, emerges from his cup of tea.[31]

Curiosity is our eagerness to find out about new things, our inquisitiveness and our sense of excitement at finding the unexpected. In 350 BCE, Aristotle introduced his Metaphysics with the statement 'All men by nature desire to know'.[32] Rene Descartes agreed: for him, our innate curiosity is an essential means of increasing knowledge.[33] Theodore Zeldin takes this argument a stage further, concluding that curiosity can be a successful remedy against sadness and fear. If we use our personal worries as stimuli to explore the general mystery of the universe, 'the limits of curiosity are at the frontiers of despair'.[34] Tolstoy (and his alter ego Levin) is a strong example of this, his profound anxiety provoking him into examining what it means to be good and do good in the world, and as a result finding a sense of peace and meaning in place of existential dread.

Imagination is our ability to produce ideas or images of what is not present or has not been experienced, and the ability to deal creatively with unexpected or unusual problems. The enhancement of memory by imagination can help us 'through the traffic jams of the brain'.[35] Imagination is at the heart of all literary activity, allowing us to recreate the world as something other than itself.[36] It is liberating when it is constructive, arranging fertile marriages between images and sensations, recombining obstacles to make them useful, spotting what is both unique and universal in them. Returning to Graham Swift's story of Jane Fairchild, we find her, with the help of the novels of Joseph Conrad, transforming herself after Paul's death from domestic servant to celebrated author.

The concept of desire refers to our innate will to persist and continue with our lives; it articulates our determination to survive, come what may. My understanding of this concept as the essence of our being derives from the *conatus* of the seventeenth-century Dutch philosopher Baruch Spinoza. He provides a compelling account of the essential coherence of the self, and in particular of our innate desire for survival, within a monist view of the world. He attributed a oneness or singleness to existence, understanding God and nature to be indistinguishable, as expressed in his phrase *Deus sive Natura* (God or nature).

Spinoza's *conatus* has variously been translated as striving, endeavour, tendency and effort and also has meanings related to power, will, appetite and desire. It is the essential attribute of all things, and in particular of human beings. It has to do with a striving towards self-maintenance:

Each thing, in so far as it is in itself, endeavours to persevere in its being.

The endeavour by which each thing endeavours to persevere in its being is nothing other than the *actual essence of the thing* (my emphasis).

The mind, both in so far as it has clear and distinct ideas and in so far as it has confused ideas, endeavours in its being for an indefinite duration, and is conscious of this endeavour.[37]

Spinoza distinguishes several aspects of *conatus*. In so far as *conatus* is related to human mind alone, it is called will (*voluntas*). When related to the mind and body simultaneously, it is called appetite (*appetitus*). In so far as humans are conscious of their appetites, Spinoza refers to them as desires (*cupiditas*). This is the term he uses most often:

> Desire is the very essence of man, in so far as it is conceived as determined to do something from some given affection of itself.[38]

Each particular thing, interacting with other particular things within the common order of nature, exhibits a characteristic tendency towards cohesion and to the preservation of its identity. All living things strive towards self-maintenance. The essence of a thing has certain necessary consequences. The thing will endeavour to persist in its own being unless it is hindered by something eternal to it; the thing has the power to persist in its own being unless impeded by external things.

Spinoza's belief in the oneness of existence, that God and nature are indistinguishable, leads him to propose intuition as specific kind of knowledge, distinct from imagination and understanding. Intuition enables us to 'proceed from an adequate idea of the formal essence of some of the attributes of God to an adequate knowledge of the essence of things'.[39] We are very close here to Duns Scotus and the 'univocity of being', and hence to the concept of inscape, the overflowing presence of the divine within the temporal, which I noted in Chapter 5 as being central to the poetic intuition of Gerard Manley Hopkins.[40] This sense of the universal being at work also informs Hopkins' understanding of his own coherence as a person, expressed most beautifully in his comments on a spiritual exercise in Liverpool in 1880:

> .. when I consider my selfbeing, my consciousness and feeling of myself, that taste of myself, of *I* and *me* above and in all things, which is more distinctive than the taste of ale or alum, more distinctive than the smell of walnutleaf or camphor, and is incommunicable by any means to another man [...] Nothing else in nature comes near this unspeakable stress of pitch, distinctiveness, and selving, this self-being of my own.[41]

Spinoza's *conatus* had a deep influence on Schopenhauer's concept of the will to life,[42] and through him an indirect impact on Tolstoy's thinking on this subject. We find Levin gaining temporary comfort from thinking he could turn his universal will into a universal love.[43] It also seems to me to be a crucial factor in the continuing life of my patient Darren.

I first met Darren as a very distressed and angry young man, aged 19, with multiple piercings and visible scars on both his arms. He did not have a lot to live for. His stories – more furious diatribes, littered with expletives – were of being caught up in the ongoing acrimony of parental separation, past experiences of emotional abuse by foster parents and relentless bullying in school. He had no qualifications, was unemployed, single and lived in a tiny flat on a busy main road with an aunt who had several long-term medical conditions. Cutting himself with a razor gave temporary relief from psychic pain. Alcohol numbed his senses but also led to fights with friends, nightclub doormen and police. His other comfort was beating the hell out of his drum kit in the middle of the night. He didn't think he'd survive much longer and didn't seem to care whether it was a deeper than usual razor cut or a harder than usual punch from a policeman that finished him off.

And yet. Darren came to see me, and kept on coming to see me. Behind his angry ranting, I heard a lost, lonely and frightened little boy. But I also saw a person with a desire to survive, to persevere in his own being. His rage against the injustices of life, particularly of his own life, was based on a deep assumption that things should not be as they were. He deserved better. He was worth more than this.

If people kill themselves out of misery, or suffer torture and death for the sake of a cause, or sacrifice themselves for the sake of their children, Spinoza argues that this is not the act of people who are independent.[44] These acts arise because they are in some way impeded from carrying out their essential self-preservative functions. Their agency is limited by the structures within which they find themselves. People living in highly adverse circumstances have their power and their choices severely constrained, sometimes to the point where non-existence may become the preferred option: those like Charlie, having experienced severe and sustained domestic violence and now, in the midst of a pandemic, being unable to contact the grandchild she loves; people forcibly transported in inhuman conditions from west Africa to the Americas to face a life of slavery[45]; or farmers in South India ground down by the relentlessly undermining effects of extreme poverty.[46] The act of suicide may become the only expression of agency left open to them.

In extreme circumstances, our sense of coherence may become overwhelmed, or disappear completely. We find Levin's sense of self-disintegrating in the face of his brother's death: unable to generate any personal meaning to his life, he is like 'a person who has traded his warm fur coat for muslin clothing and, caught in the cold for the first time, is convinced [he.....] must inevitably die a painful death'[47]. We witness Hopkins' 'cliffs of fall/ Frightful, sheer, no-man-fathomed', where his only relief is that thought that 'all/ Life death does end and each day dies with sleep'.[48] And Darren's sense of self was, quite literally, on a knife's edge.

Vastly More Intersubjectivity

Our sense of identity has essential social dimensions. I cannot be a self on my own. Realising this is sometimes essential to our survival.

The second component of my concept of the self is the assumption that we make sense of ourselves and find meaning in our engagement with the world around us: in the context of the history, places or 'practices' within which we find ourselves, and which we have the ability to modify; and within this, a belief that such engagement – whether constructed in political, social, spiritual or personal terms – is crucial in creating our sense of identity and well-being. Our engagement may be active, in the sense of our positively choosing to be involved in the world around us; it also contains reactive or receptive elements, including allowing ourselves to be cared for by others, to have our own basic needs met.

Reflecting on ways to ease the fragmenting effects of dementia, but with insights that apply equally to the isolating experience of suicide, Tom Kitwood and Kathleen Bredin propose that personhood 'should be viewed as essentially social: it refers to the human being in relation to others'. They see interdependence as a necessary condition of being human:

> A more desirable form of life would be one in which there was vastly more intersubjectivity, and where there would be a continuing opportunity for people to be fluid; or, to alter the image, to grow and change.[49]

At the level of political philosophy, this position is supported by John Milbank and Adrian Pabst in their argument for a civil economy within which the rights of the individual are blended with principles of reciprocity and mutuality.[50] And from an anthropological perspective, Ludek Brodz and Daniel Münster remind us that the discrete self is a particularly Western liberal notion, and that in many other cultures, 'humans are seen not as bounded subjects, whose behaviour is influenced, shaped or determined by social structures or bio-medical mechanisms, but as extended or distributed beyond the individual'.[51] Beatriz Reyes-Foster, reflecting on the suicides of two young women in Yucatan, Mexico, notes the fluidity of boundaries between the Yucatecan person and the space they occupy, and that 'the self is not merely one part of the community; rather the entire community is a system of selves connected in space and time'.[52]

Engagement may take the form of participation in practices and moral communities, defined by Alasdair MacIntyre as 'coherent and complex form of socially established cooperative human activity' with inherent standards of excellence.[53] In this sense, it is closely related to the Greek term *eudaemonia*, which encompasses both being well and doing well, the expectation of acting not only for oneself but for purposes beyond oneself, making choices that lead to right action.[54]

Practices involve the use of a set of skills in a systematic way, with the intention of enriching our lives and the lives of those around us. Practices may be self-contained, for example playing chess or music, experimenting with the structure of the sonnet (for Gerard Manley Hopkins) or keeping bees (for Leo Tolstoy and Levin). Practices may also be purposive, such as law and politics, general medical practice or writing a book about how literary reading may help people decide to stay alive.

Moral communities involve friendship within common pursuit of purposes beyond oneself, such as the political community of classical Athens, medieval monastic orders and the liberation movements in late twentieth century Africa. In my own case, moral communities with friendships and common pursuits include two long-term European research groups and the World Organisation of Family Doctors' working party for mental health. And in *A Long Way Down*, Nick Hornby creates a moral community in the self-help group formed by Martin, Maureen, JJ and Jess.

Engagement may also take the simpler form, proposed by Charles Taylor, of the affirmation of ordinary life through investment in our networks. This involves reference to a defining community, which may be narrow, spatial or broad; intellectual, religious, political or national; and which may include both the living and dead. I am a self in relation to my conversation partners, who are crucial to my continuing grasp of self-understanding. I cannot be a self on my own. My self exists within 'webs of interlocution':

> I define who I am by defining where I speak from, in the family tree, in social space, in the geography of social statuses and functions, in my intimate relations to the ones I love, and also crucially in the space of moral and spiritual orientation within which my most important defining relations are lived out.[55]

For Constantin Levin and Gerard Manley Hopkins, investing in their networks, engaging with their webs of interlocution, saves them from self-destruction, and enables them to rediscover or create their reasons to be. Levin immerses himself in the practical work of managing his country estate, his daily interactions with Kitty, his family and friends, and arranging a washstand for his baby son. Throughout his darkest days in Dublin, Hopkins maintains regular correspondence with his close friend Robert Bridges, can 'Kind love both give and get' in interactions with his family in England and the people he meets in University College, and (for him most importantly) finds eventual comfort in his God 'whose smile [....] as skies/Betweenpie mountains – lights a lovely mile'.[56]

Darren comes to see me every few weeks over the next few years. He stays alive. It is fair to assume that, for quite a while, our regular 10- or 15-minute conversations are a crucial investment in his otherwise very precarious network, one of the few (perhaps the only) positive elements in his defining community. He still mostly rants, and I still mostly listen, but there are less alcohol and fewer fights in his life. His web of interlocution gradually expands. He rescues an Alsatian dog who he renames Koda, a Sioux word meaning friend, companion or ally. They become inseparable. He takes a music course at a local college to improve his drumming skills and through this finds a place with two local bands, one with a possible recording contract. He starts a relationship with Mark, bass guitarist in one of these bands. who lives with him on and off. He helps his younger brother separate from the baleful influence of their mother and even supports his father through a complicated psychiatric emergency admission. Beneath the anguish, there is a young man with a keen critical intelligence, compassion for his family and friends and disdain for rhetorical 'political bullshit'. We have some lively conversations about epistemic injustice and existentialism. He is keen to follow up on the writings of Miranda Fricker and becomes intrigued by Jean-Paul Sartre's *Road to Freedom* trilogy. Like Mathieu Delarue, he is determined to live his life genuinely, authentically, whatever the cost.

The Struggle towards the Heights

Engagement may also take the form of commitment to the circumstances in which we find ourselves, whatever they may be, whether they involve cultural alienation or physical illness, and our determination to make of them the best we can. Our role model here is the boulder-pushing Sisyphus, as interpreted by Albert Camus. For Camus, the key philosophical question is whether the conflict between our human need for understanding and the meaninglessness and absurdity of life necessarily leads us to consider suicide.

> There is but one truly serious philosophical problem, and that is suicide. Judging whether life is or is not worth living amounts to answering the fundamental question of philosophy.

He is keeping company here with practically everyone we have met in this book: with Al Alvarez and his contemporaries, with Tolstoy and Levin, with Hopkins and Schopenhauer. Like them, Camus ultimately rejects suicide as an option, though his reasoning and his response are different. He agrees with Spinoza and Schopenhauer that we have an irrepressible will to live: 'in a man's attachment to life there is something stronger than all the ills in the world'. The contradiction between the desire of human reason and an unreasonable world must be lived.

> The real effort is to stay there, rather, in so far as that is possible, and to examine closely the odd vegetation of those distant regions. Tenacity and acumen are privileged spectators of this inhuman show in which absurdity, hope, and death carry on their dialogue[57].

We must embrace all that the world has to offer, in a spirit of revolt, freedom and passion. Whether like Charlie we experience daily oppression through our destructive intimate relationships, or like Hopkins and Darren we find ourselves in a place of profound social and political alienation, or whether are facing existential threat through a combination of accelerating climate change and a global pandemic, the conclusion is the same. We must resist. We must live.

> Consciousness and revolt, these rejections are the contrary of renunciation. Everything that is indomitable and passionate in a human heart quickens them, on the contrary, with its own life. It is essential to die unreconciled and not of one's own free will. Suicide is a repudiation. The absurd man can only drain everything to the bitter end, and deplete himself. The absurd is his extreme tension, which he maintains constantly by solitary effort, for he knows that in that consciousness and in that day-to-day revolt he gives proof of his only truth, which is defiance[58].

Sisyphus is for ever straining to push his rock up the hill before watching it roll all the way back down again. In Camus' interpretation, his happiness is inseparable from the absurd situation in which he finds himself. He knows that there is no ultimate logical or purpose in what he is doing, but this gives him a sense of liberation rather than oppression. He chooses to do what he is doing. He is happy because his fate belongs to him. He remains his own master, his mind and body fully engaged in his chosen activity:

> I leave Sisyphus at the foot of the mountain. One always finds one's burden again. But Sisyphus teaches the higher fidelity that negates the gods and raises rocks. He too concludes that all is well. This universe henceforth without a master seems to him neither sterile nor futile. Each atom of that stone, each mineral flake of that night filled mountain, in itself forms a world. The struggle itself toward the heights is enough to fill a man's heart[59].

Recently, Darren's life has become more difficult again. He disagrees with the musical direction of the band with the recording contract, and they have parted company. He has money worries and is involved with endless arguments with the benefits agency. His partner is still around, but Mark has a lot of problems of his own and they are finding it difficult to get along together.

Then, Koda dies, run over by a careless driver on the road outside his flat.

Darren is devastated, grieving inconsolably for one of the very few sentient beings with whom he has ever enjoyed a mutually supportive relationship. He feels he is back to where he was a decade ago, not caring whether he lives or dies. He is cutting himself again, now on his thighs, and drinking a lot more alcohol. He spends most of the day lying on bed. He cannot even find the energy to play his drums. I am very concerned that his defining community, even though less precarious than it was, will not be sufficiently robust to persuade him to stay alive. For several months, it is touch and go.

But Darren does keep coming to see me, and Mark is able to put his own problems aside sufficiently to offer him the unconditional support he needs. Gradually, he pulls through. His rage against the machine, which we both now recognise as his motivating force, begins to kick back into life. He resumes his warrior role, this time on behalf of his aunt's rejected social security claims.

Like Camus, his response to the absurdities of his life is one of passionate rebellion. He finishes Sartre's trilogy and is fascinated by Mathieu's final stand in the village clocktower, facing death at the hands of the advancing enemy but determined to end with an uncompromising, ecstatic act of freedom:

> Nothing more to ask of Fate now except one half-minute. Just enough time to fire at that smart officer, at all the Beauty of the Earth, at the street, at the flowers, at the gardens, at everything he had loved. Beauty dived downwards like some obscene bird. But Mathieu went on firing. He fired. He was cleansed. He was all-powerful, He was free[60].

'Fuck yes' Darren tells me, 'I'd fucking totally be up for that!'. I want to offer him a high-five or a fist-bump, but feel inhibited by my professional position and the current pandemic regulations. Instead, I just smile behind my face-mask. It occurs to me later that his authenticity is in better shape than mine.

Continually Completely New?

In this chapter, I have reviewed and suggested a variety of philosophical sources in a quest to find *raisons d'etre* for people who are facing a dilemma about their continued existence, or for those who are supporting and caring for them. I have noted – without much enthusiasm – Hamlet's worries about facing something worse than life in death, and the deontological position that it is our obligation, our moral duty to live the life we have been given. I have shown how Kierkegaard, like Tolstoy and Hopkins, understands religious belief to be the fundamental *raison d'etre*. I have given support to the views of Schopenhauer and Spinoza that we have an innate will to life, a desire to persevere in our existences, which carries us through tough times, especially when our own suffering creates a sense of compassion for the distress of others. When our sense of coherence is threatened, our intersubjective engagement with others, whether in the form of moral communities or webs of interlocution, can be a powerful antidote to despair. And we may find with Camus that acknowledging the absurdity of life generates in us an energetic spirit of revolt, passion and freedom.

A final philosophical reflection, courtesy of Galen Strawson. What if our sense of a coherent self is not, actually, real; what if there is a disconnect between our phenomenological experience of the world and its metaphysical or ontological facts? In his seminal book, *Selves*, Strawson combines rigorous analytical philosophy with the central tenet of Buddhist no-self to propose that, while we may perceive ourselves to exist continuously and assume ourselves to be (in his terms) single subjects of experience, this coherence dissolves in the face of our inner mental subjectivity.

> I feel I have continuity through the waking day only as an embodied human being [......] When I consider myself in the whole-human-being way I fully endorse the conventional view that there is in my case – that I am – a single subject of experience – a person – with long-term diachronic continuity. But when I experience myself as an inner mental subject and consider the detailed character of conscious experience, my feeling is that I am – that the thing that I most essentially am is – continually completely new.[61]

Strawson argues instead towards the concept of 'thin' selves, which may be many and transient. He is in favour of the idea that we find many short-lived subjects of experience, even when we consider a single human being. He gives the example of Louis as a representative human being, who is a short-lived subject of the present moment, for example while admiring the internal architecture of St Paul's cathedral in London. We could also recast Tim Bayne's description of his Cuban café visit as that of a thin-self subject of experience. These multiple thin selves are coherent entities in their own right, each experiencing, being a subject and having some content. But they do not have a necessary connection with the selves that existed before them or will come into being after them.

Strawson is not advocating a state of total existential anarchy. He believes Spinoza to be fundamentally correct in asserting the reality of human subjectivity within the one subject of experience, the universe: we are not individual objects but rather features, modes or modifications of the only object there is, the universe: 'it is true that there is diversity but also true that it is, somehow, all one'.[62] So we are still in the realms of inter-subjectivity and univocity, now extended to our relationships with ourselves as well as with other sentient beings, and (like Hopkin's inscape) with our environment on the earth and beyond: the whole system as a single, complex, inter-related organism.[63]

For me, Strawson's multiple selves, his sense of being continually and completely new, are exciting and liberating. We are not necessarily and irretrievably trapped within any particular way of viewing the world or our own positions within it. Perhaps one day, like Raimund Gregorius, I board the night train for Lisbon[64] (or Paris, or Prague) and discover an entirely different version of the many lives I could have lived. Perhaps Darren becomes a civil rights activist or a local politician. Perhaps, his drumming skills are rewarded with a recording contract.

Our selves are neither fixed nor determined. We exist, but with the perpetual potential to change, to grow and to flourish.

Notes

1 Arthur Schopenhauer, *The World as Will and Representation: Volume 2*, trans. Eric Payne (New York: Dover, 1969), 634, 637.

2 Arthur Schopenhauer, *Paregra and Paralipomena: Short Philosophical Essays*, trans. Eric Payne (Oxford: Clarendon, 1974), 294.

3 Schopenhauer, *Paregra*, ibid., 298–99.

4 Søren Kierkegaard, *The Sickness unto Death* (Princeton: Princeton University Press, 1983), 45.

5 David Benatar, *Better Never to Have Been: The Harm of Coming into Existence* (Oxford: Clarendon Press, 2006).

6 Len Doyal, 'Is Human Existence Worth Its Consequent Harm?' *Journal of Medical Ethics* 33, no. 10 (2007): 573–76.

7 Schopenhauer, *World as Will and Representation: Volume 1*, ibid., 398–99.

8 Gregory Maertz. 'Elective Affinities: Tolstoy and Schopenhauer'. *Wiener Slavistisches Jahrbuch* 40 (1994): 53–62.

9 Schopenhauer, *World as Will and Representation: Volume 1*, ibid., 399.

10 Andrew Bennett, *Suicide Century* (Cambridge: Cambridge University Press, 2017), 36.

11 Schopenhauer, *World as Will and Representation: Volume 1*, ibid., 68.

12 Timothy Madigan, 'Schopenhauer's Compassionate Morality'. *Philosophy Now*, 2005, https://philosophynow.org/issues/52/Schopenhauers_Compassionate_Morality. Accessed 13 May 2021.

13 Arthur Schopenhauer, *Essays and Aphorisms*, trans. Reginald Hollingdale (London: Penguin Books, 1970), 50.

14 Søren Kierkegaard, *The Soul of Kierkegaard: Selections from His Journal*, ed. Alexander Dru (New York: Dover Publications, 2003), 236.

15 Kierkegaard, *Sickness unto Death*, ibid.

16 Walpola Rahula, *What the Buddha Taught* (Oxford: Oneworld Publications, 1959), 93.

17 Christopher Dowrick, *Beyond Depression* (Oxford: Oxford University Press, 2009), 54.

18 Gananeth Obeyesekere, 'Depression, Buddhism, and the Work of Culture in Sri Lanka', in *Culture and Depression: Studies in the Anthropology and Cross-Cultural Psychiatry of Affect and Disorder*, ed. Arthur Kleinman and Byron Good (Berkeley: University of California Press, 1985), 134–52.

19 Jonardon Ganeri, *The Self* (Oxford: Oxford University Press, 2012).

20 Ronald Epstein, *Attending: Medicine, Mindfulness and Humanity* (New York: Scribner, 2017).

21 Karl Barth, *Church Dogmatics III/2*, 2nd edition, trans. Harold Knight et al., eds. Geoffrey Bromiley and Thomas Torrance (Peabody, MA: Hendrickson, 2010).

22 Martin Buber, *I and Thou*, ed. and trans. Walter Kaufmann (New York: Touchstone, 1970).

23 Ronald Epstein, 'Whole Mind and Shared Mind in Clinical Decision-Making'. *Patient Education and Counselling* 90, no. 2 (2013): 200–06.

24 Dowrick, Beyond *Depression*, ibid., 59–197.

25 Christopher Dowrick, 'Suffering, Meaning and Hope' in *Sadness or Depression?* ed. Jerome Wakefield and Steeves Demazeux (Dordrecht: Springer, 2016), 121–36.

26 Christopher Dowrick, 'Patient, Person, Self', in *Person-Centred Primary Care*, ed. Christopher Dowrick (London: Routledge, 2018), 119–40.

27 Elizabeth Anscombe, *Intention* (Cambridge: Harvard University Press, 2000).

28 Tim Bayne, *The Unity of Consciousness* (Oxford: Oxford University Press, 2010), 5.

29 Bayne, *Unity of Consciousness*, ibid., 289–94.

30 Richard Wollheim, *The Thread of Life* (Cambridge: Cambridge University Press, 1984).

31 Marcel Proust, *In Search of Lost Time. Volume 1: Swann's Way*, trans. Charles Scott Moncrieff et al. (London: Vintage Press, 2002), 51–55.

32 William Ross, *Aristotle's Metaphysics* (Oxford: Clarendon Press, 1953).

33 Rene Descartes, 'Treatise on the Passions of the Soul', in *Philosophical Works Of Descartes*, trans. Elizabeth Halden and George Ross (Cambridge: Cambridge University Press, 1967).

34 Theodore Zeldin, *An Intimate History of Humanity* (London: Sinclair-Stevenson, 1994), 202.

35 Zeldin, *Intimate History*, ibid., 441–42.

36 Bennett, *Suicide Century*, ibid., 34.

37 Baruch Spinoza, *Ethics*, ed. and trans. George Parkinson (Oxford: Oxford University Press, 2000): part III, Propositions 6, 7 and 9.

38 Spinoza, *Ethics*, ibid.: Part III, Definitions of Emotions.

39 Spinoza, *Ethics*, ibid., 149.

40 Joshua Hall, 'Poetic Imagination: Spinoza and Gerard Manley Hopkins'. *Philosophy Today* 57 (2013): 401–07.

41 Gerard Manley Hopkins, 'Comments on the Spiritual Exercises of St. Ignatius Loyola', in *Poems and Prose of Gerard Manley Hopkins*, ed. William Gardner (London: Penguin Books, 1968), 145–46.

42 Henry Brann, 'Schopenhauer and Spinoza', *Journal of the History of Philosophy* 10, no. 2 (1972): 181–96.

43 Leo Tolstoy, *Anna Karenina*, trans. Richard Pevear and Larissa Volokhonsky (London: Penguin Books 2003), 788.

44 Steven Nadler, 'Spinoza on Lying and Suicide', *British Journal for the History of Philosophy* 24, no. 2 (2016): 257–78.

45 Katy Ryan, 'Revolutionary Suicide in Toni Morrison's Fiction'. *African American Review* 34, no. 3 (2000): 389–412.

46 Daniel Münster, 'Farmers' Suicide and the Moral Economy of Agriculture', in *Suicide and Agency*, eds. Ludek Broz and Daniel Münster (London: Routledge, 2020), 105–25.

47 Tolstoy, *Anna Karenina*, ibid., 786.

48 Hopkins, 'No Worst, There is None' in *Poems and Prose*, ibid., 61.

49 Tom Kitwood and Kathleen Bredin, 'Towards a Theory of Dementia Care: Personhood and Wellbeing'. *Ageing and Society* 12, no. 3 (1992): 269–87.

50 John Millbank and Adrian Pabst, *The Politics of Virtue* (Lanham: Rowman and Littlefield, 2016).

51 Daniel Münster and Ludek Broz, 'The Anthropology of Suicide: Ethnography and the Tension of Agency', in *Suicide and Agency*, ibid., 15.

52 Beatriz Reyes-Foster, 'Between Demons and Disease: Suicide and Agency in Yucatan, Mexico', in *Suicide and Agency*, ibid., 75.

53 Alasdair MacIntyre, *After Virtue: A Study in Moral Theory*, 2nd edition (Notre Dame Indiana: University of Notre Dame Press, 1984), 187.

54 Aristotle. *The Nichomachean Ethics*, trans. William Ross et al. (Oxford: Oxford Paperbacks, 1998).

55 Charles Taylor, *Sources of the Self: The Making of the Modern Identity* (Cambridge: Cambridge University Press, 1989), 35.

56 Hopkins, 'To Seem the Stranger' and 'My Own Heart' in *Poems and Prose*, ibid., 62, 63.

57 Albert Camus, *The Myth of Sisyphus and Other Essays*, trans. Justin O'Brien. (New York: Vintage Books, 1991), 9.

58 Camus, *Myth of Sisyphus*, ibid., 55.

59 Camus, *Myth of Sisyphus*, ibid., 123.

60 Jean Paul Sartre, *Iron in the Soul*, trans. Gerard Hopkins (London: Penguin Books, 1963), 225.

61 Galen Strawson, *Selves: An Essay in Revisionary Metaphysics* (Oxford: Oxford University Press, 2009), 247.

62 Strawson, *Selves*, ibid., 424.

63 James Lovelock and Lynn Margulis, L. 'Atmospheric Homeostasis by and for the Biosphere: The Gaia hypothesis'. *Tellus* 26, nos. 1–2 (1974): 2–10.

64 Pascal Mercier P., *Night Train to Lisbon*, trans. Barbara Harshaw (London: Atlantic Books, 2008).

Chapter 7

STAYING ALIVE

It has been my intention in this book to explore the ways in which literary reading can help people who are contemplating suicide decide to stay alive. I have also sought to demonstrate how literary reading can interact with theoretical perspectives from social psychology and philosophy to enhance our understanding of the suicidal experience.

Using evidence from epidemiological and literary sources, including the World Health Organisation and James Joyce, I have shown that suicidal thoughts and actions are common occurrences. I have discussed a range of sociological, psychological and anthropological theories explaining why people consider ending their lives, interweaving these together with the substantial literary testimonies of Leo Tolstoy, with particular focus on the characters of Anna Karenina and Konstantin Levin, and with the poetic insights of Gerard Manley Hopkins. I have linked these with my own experiences and those of patients whom it has been my privilege to encounter; all the while acknowledging, with Anna Karenina, my patient Charlie and David Foster Wallace, the unresolvable uncertainties around the inevitability or otherwise of the suicidal act.

With the help of Tolstoy and Hopkins, ably supported by Al Alvarez and Stevie Smith, I have explored direct personal experiences of facing the dilemma of existence and how ending one's life can appear to be the only viable option. And with Tolstoy's particular insights, I have imagined with Anna Karenina what the last few moments of life might actually be like.

I have reflected on the question of why people in the depths of despair might consider staying alive and found a wide variety of responses, ranging from Hamlet's fear that death may be even worse, through the conviction of Alvarez and Schopenhauer that suicide provides us with no answers, to the sense of compassion – for self and others – which (eventually) radiates through the poetics of Hopkins and emerges in the philosophy of Schopenhauer. I have noted how Hopkins' determination to survive is reflected in the *conatus* of Spinoza and how even the deeply ambivalent Stevie

Smith encourages us to keep on keeping on. I have shown how Peter Porter and Seamus Heaney have chosen to confront and challenge the seriousness of living and considered Matt Haig's literary and Galen Strawson's philosophical reflections on the infinite possibilities of existence. And I have suggested that people bereaved by suicide, like Jane Goodchild and my patient Leigh, may still thrive.

In the process of considering who or what may help us to stay alive, I have commended Tolstoy's and Levin's approach to 'doing' rather than 'thinking', and Hopkins' emerging sense of self-compassion. I have explored ways in which we can increase our social connectedness, our intersubjectivity: through engagement with family, like Egil Skallagrimsson and his daughter Torgedur; with friends, like Kitty and Varenka, or the Toppers' House self-help group; or through a supportive relationship with an ancient Egyptian Ba or (failing that) a sympathetic health professional. Our engagement may also take the form of seeking to do good in the world, though not necessarily with the scale and ambition of Tolstoy. For some, like Tolstoy and Hopkins, in company with Kierkegaard, reasons to stay alive may emerge through belief in a greater spiritual good; or like Hopkins again, this time in company of Duns Scotus and Spinoza, through a sense of the oneness, the universal interconnectedness of being. Or we may decide to follow Albert Camus in his defiant, passionate rebellion against the absurdity of our existence.

Sunt Lacrimae Rerum

In my first chapter I indicated that therapeutic strategies in relation to suicide have three main purposes: increasing a sense of hope, reducing the power of suicidal thoughts and maximising the power of the individual not to act on them. It seems to me that literary reading can have impact in all of these domains.

The specific advantage of literary reading is that it builds on and then moves beyond the reach of social psychology and philosophy, entering into the confusing and chaotic heart of the suicidal experience in ways that even the profoundest theoretical insights are unable to do. Engaging with Tolstoy or Hopkins, Joyce or Smith, Hornby or Haig, or so many others, we are transported to places which are simultaneously real and not real, where the combination of the 'otherness' and brilliance of the novel or the poem allows us the space, and at the same time gives us the courage, to acknowledge the deeply unconsolable, to engage with the inadmissible, to hold thoughts and experience emotions which we would otherwise fear it would almost kill us to contain.[1]

For people considering suicide, like my teenage self and my patient Frances, literary reading provides an awareness that we are not alone, which can be of great significance given the intense sense of isolation and alienation that often form part of the suicidal experience. It begins to expand opportunities for us to exercise our self-compassion and self-forgiveness, which a recent systematic review has shown are strongly associated with a reduction in suicidal ideation and self-harm.[2] And it offers us alternative scenarios and solutions to the dilemma of our existence, as with Frances' mindful walking and Darren's civic activism.

For those of us caring for people considering suicide, whether family, friends or health professionals, literary reading extends our sense of compassion, allowing us 'the possibility of imagining suicide and of feeling empathy towards individuals who undertake it'.[3] It enables us to overcome that first, sometimes immense hurdle, composed of a combination of ego-centricity, uncertainty, confusion and dread, which 'closes off compassion and stops us from being healers'.[4] We become more able to turn towards suffering, become more curious about the person's experience and intentionally become more present and engaged.[5] With the result that we can simply, and crucially, sit with and listen to the person in despair.

Bearing witness to suffering, giving the other person a sense of being understood and accepted, is the first essential step towards hope.

This thought brings me to my final literary extract, this time Virgil's Latin epic poem *The Aeneid*, composed between 29 and 19 BCE and commended to me a few years ago by my classically educated mother. In the first book, we find Aeneas as a refugee, making his weary way to Italy, driven far from home by the vicious ravages of the Trojan War. He is in Carthage, gazing at a mural in a temple, which depicts battles of the Trojan War and the deaths of many of his friends and countrymen. He is moved to tears and offers a rousing tribute to his fallen comrades:

Sunt hic etiam sua praemia laudi; sunt lacrimae rerum et mentem mortalia tangunt.
Solve metus; feret haec aliquam tibi fama salutem.[6]
    [Here too the praiseworthy has its rewards; there are tears of/for things and mortal things touch the mind. Release your fear; this fame will bring you some safety.]

It's just three words – *sunt lacrimae rerum* – that I want to concentrate on: this phrase brings us to the heart of the link between suffering and hope.

Rerum is the genitive of *res* (things) and, importantly, can be understood in both objective and subjective terms. So this phrase has been translated as either 'there are tears for things' or else 'there are tears of things'. The first, objective version indicates the burdens we have to bear, the frailty of human existence and the 'shit life syndrome' so many people experience. The second, subjective version indicates that things feel sorrow for our suffering – that in some sense the universe feels our pain.

But of course, it is not one or the other. It is both. Virgil is fully aware of the ambiguity and wishes to us to understand both meanings at the same time. So does Seamus Heaney, who translates the phrase as 'There are tears at the heart of things'.[7]

And this is its richness and power. At that moment when I experience and express compassion for the suffering of the person in the room with me, both senses of *sunt lacrimae rerum* are simultaneously in play. They can express pain, distress and suffering, knowing that – from me – they find understanding, compassion and safety. Our meeting place has become, momentarily, a sanctuary.[8]

This is exactly what people in the deepest distress want. US military veterans who were diagnosed with serious mental illness and had attempted suicide were asked for their views about the best ways to improve their care. Their most common recommendation was to increase the empathy, compassion and listening skills of the clinicians who were attending them. They were 'yearning to be heard'.[9]

And compassion has demonstrable benefits in practice. A Dutch observational study of 348 patients with depression in primary care found that an accurate diagnosis of depression and adequate antidepressant treatment was associated with better patient outcomes, including reduced suicidal ideation, but only when provided by supportive and empathic general practitioners.[10] A series of studies in Scotland have shown how patients' perceptions of their clinician's empathy are key to their sense of enablement, their sense of feeling empowered after a consultation, in terms of being able to cope with, understand and manage their illness[11] and that this sense of enablement in turn is crucial in leading to improvement in symptom severity and related well-being.[12]

When the time is right for that person (not too soon, and not merely to ease our own vicarious distress), we can indicate how literary reading offers alternative ways of looking at the world, new possibilities for hope. We may wish to introduce literary reference directly into our conversations or consultations, as I have shown in my encounters with Frances and Darren. Sometimes the literary flow is in the other direction: for example, I was introduced to Matt Haig's *Midnight Library* by a depressed – and previously suicidal – patient who found it inspiring and hopeful and wanted to share the benefits with me.

We can readily incorporate this approach within existing strategies designed to reduce the likelihood of people acting on their suicidal thoughts. Let us take the example of the New Economics Foundation's *Five Ways to Wellbeing*. These are summarised as Connect, Be Active, Take Notice, Learn and Give, and are promoted as valuable ways of improving our individual and collective mental health.[13] The encouragement of literary reading can have a direct mitigating influence on the suicidal experience through least three of these elements. It enables healing connection between the text and the distressed person, as we have seen most clearly in the case of Frances; and if taking place in a reading group it also leads to therapeutic connections between the group members, as I explained in the first chapter.[14] Intrinsically, it encourages the reader to take notice, to become more aware of the real and imagined worlds around them, to remark on the new and, perhaps keeping company with Hopkins and his Windhover, to catch sight of the beautiful. And literary reading also offers us multiple, potentially infinite opportunities for learning about new things, from bee-keeping in nineteenth century Russia to theories of parallel universes.

Or we may consider our personal reading of literature and poetry as an additional and entirely legitimate source of our own wisdom, adding to whatever trove of scientific, clinical philosophical or experiential knowledge we already possess, and in so doing increasing our capacity to act as catalysts for or reagents with others in their process of transformation away from death and towards life. I can bring to mind Kitty's ridiculous medical consultations as an antidote to the perils of medical pomposity and reflect on Levin's wholehearted engagement in his customary pursuits when explaining the benefits of doing things that bring a sense of enjoyment or accomplishment, without having to discuss them with the person in distress. I do not have to quote Hopkins' 'not choose not to be' or Keats' 'No go not to Lethe' when helping someone on the verge of suicide decide that survival may after all be possible. Simply having these reservoirs of knowledge, these inspirations to draw on is often entirely sufficient.

And for those bereaved by suicide, like Leigh, literary reading offers relief through acknowledgement of its inexplicability (and hence reduction in any sense of responsibility or guilt), and through the gradual emergence of the awareness that a fulfilling life afterwards is, nevertheless, possible. Reflecting now as I write, I realise for the first time that this applies to me too in relation to my reactions to the death of Charlie. I have become aware of my own sense of guilt and regret that I did not do enough to protect her during the maelstrom that tormented the final days her life. My observations about her parallel universes may bring more comfort to me than to her.

Back to Black

I am not intending to claim that literary reading is the only way in which our sense of (self-) compassion, our belief and hope in the possibility of alternative responses to the dilemma of existence may be fostered and encouraged. If Aristotelian catharsis is at the heart of literature's ability to generate change, it is surely also to be found in other artistic endeavours, whether in the form of the visual or the performing arts.

If I were looking for paintings that best portray the three people whose stories have illuminated this book, I might begin with Francis Bacon's *Study for a Portrait*, with his distressed, alienated subject enclosed in the wretched Nietzschean glass capsule of the human individual,[15] as a graphic representation of Darren's anger and anguish. For Frances, I would choose Edward Hopper's *Automat*, with its neatly dressed lonely woman, staring into a cup of coffee, behind her the night stretching endlessly into the distance.[16] And Bertha Wegmann's *Despair*, with its deeply compassionate image of a woman to whom something awful has happened, leaving her in a position of utterly exhausted defeat,[17] would be a fitting representation of Charlie's final days.

If I had to choose just one illustrative piece for the themes of this book from across the world of sculpture, it would probably be Auguste Rodin's *Clenched Left Hand*, described by a curator at the New York Met as one of his 'most compelling depictions of powerless despair'.[18] I would also note the recent arrival in Bristol, United Kingdom, of a figure sitting on a high wall, head in hands, being comforted by a teddy bear.[19] The anonymous sculptor has, it appears, created this work explicitly to encourage people to talk about suicide.

There are whole worlds of suicidal imaginations to be explored in ballet, perhaps most famously in *Giselle* and *Swan Lake*,[20] and more recently Matthew Bourne's *The Red Shoes*, with its ending highly reminiscent of Anna Karenina as Victoria Page falls under an oncoming train. And even more in opera: think of Romeo in Gounod's *Romeo et Juliette* and Cio-Cio-San in Puccini's *Madama Butterfly*. Saxby Pridmore and colleagues have analysed depictions of suicide in 337 operas created over 400 years between 1607 and 2006. They find evidence of completed suicide, non-fatal suicidal acts and suicidal thoughts in 112 (33 per cent), with completed suicide being the most common, occurring in 74 (22 per cent) of all these operas. They note that these suicidal events always follow an undesirable event or situation, that cutting is the most common method and that – in a reversal of reality – men are more commonly depicted as engaging in non-fatal events whereas women are more commonly portrayed as completers.[21] There is a great deal of scope for further study and reflection here.

If classical music were my focus rather than literary reading, I would undoubtedly choose Ludwig van Beethoven as one of my original case studies. I might well begin with his Heiligenstadt Testament, a letter written to his brothers on 6 October 1802 and found in his papers after his death. In this letter, he expressed his despair over his increasing deafness and directly confronted his own dilemma of existence: on the one hand, stating that he was contemplating suicide; and on the other hand, expressing his continued desire to overcome his physical and emotional difficulties, in the hope that he could complete his artistic destiny.

Amongst his subsequent works, I would certainly explore the hauntingly beautiful *largo* from his violin concerto, perhaps the 1992 performance by Itzhak Perlman and Daniel Barenboim with the Berlin Philharmonic,[22] whose significance for me is as the sublime musical equivalent of Gerard Manley Hopkin's *The Windhover.* I would include the *molto adagio-andante* from his 15th String Quartet, written in thanksgiving for his recovery after a prolonged, near-fatal intestinal disorder and described by T. S. Eliot as 'the fruit of reconciliation and relief after immense suffering'.[23] And I would attempt (though almost certainly fail) to make sense of the magnificent pandemonium of his *Große Fuge*, with its apocalyptic struggle (to me highly prescient of Albert Camus in the face of absurdity) to overcome chaos and enable a meaningful life to evolve.[24]

Moving to (more) contemporary music, my choice of the titles of the opening and this closing chapter was prompted by the BeeGees disco classic *Stayin' Alive.* In sharp contrast to its upbeat tempo, the lyrics portray dance as a desperate act of survival, they are a plea for help from a man who has been kicked around since the day he was born, his life going nowhere. For Barry Gibb, the song was about

> People crying out for help. [....] Everybody struggles against the world, fighting all the bullshit and things that can drag you down. And it really is a victory just to survive.[25]

Looking for songs appropriate to my principal characters, I have already suggested the connections between Frances and the Beatles' *Eleanor Rigby.* And there can be few performances more evocative either of Charlie's devastated hopelessness than Amy Whitehouse's *Back to Black*, or of Darren's existential rage than Black Sabbath's *Sabbath Bloody Sabbath.*

If I were to choose a contemporary musician to join Beethoven and replace Tolstoy and Hopkins, it would probably be Bruce Springsteen, working through periods of depression and suicidal thoughts as he strove to create an identity distinct from the 'lifeless, sucking black hole' that was his childhood.[26] I would explore the catharsis for him – as for me and countless others – of riding his suicide machine in *Born to Run*; the realisation that, sometimes, anything is better than worrying about your little world falling apart, even if it's just *Dancing in the Dark*; and his reflections on the personal transformations that await us if we have the courage to explore the *Darkness on the Edge of Town*.

I am sure by now you will have many other ideas and suggestions about the ways in which a whole range of artistic endeavours can help us to confront the dilemma of existence. I would love to hear about them.

Final Reflections

Frances continues her mindful walking through the streets of Liverpool. She has survived the loss of her civil service job and, a few months later, the death of her beloved cat Danny: she has his photograph on her mantelpiece, next to a casket containing his ashes. She is still involved with her church and a support to her various friends and has become a little more willing to share her own feelings and needs with them. She has signed up as a regular volunteer in a local animal sanctuary. She is now exploring Hopkins' pastoral poetry, with *Pied Beauty* and *God's Grandeur* her current favourites. Darren remains an advocate-warrior on behalf of his family and friends. He has moved on from Sartre to James Baldwin and is newly energised by Owen Jones' articles on civil liberties in the Guardian. He has realised that his scope for effective action will be extended by working with others and has joined the Citizens Advice Bureau to campaign for changes to unfair policies and practices.

I started writing this book from the position of an academic general practitioner with a concern for patients experiencing the darkest of times. But the further I have advanced into reading, reflecting and writing, the more I have realised that I am not merely a sympathetic observer or supporter. I am also writing for and about myself as a human being, reflecting on my past and current existential concerns. I still grieve for Charlie, whether or not she is away exploring other galaxies, and regret the unimaginable distress of her final days on this earth. Anna's 'anxieties, deceptions, grief and evil', Hopkins' 'cliffs of fall, frightful, sheer no-man fathomed' are as real for me as they are for Tolstoy and Hopkins, or for Charlie, Frances and Darren. So too are the shoots of hope that emerge when Levin just starts doing what he is doing and Hopkins calls off thoughts awhile to leave comfort root-room. And the moments of joy to be found watching a falcon in flight, or arranging a washstand for a new-born baby.

I hope that some of these reflections have also been of benefit to you.

Notes

1 Josie Billington, *Is Literature Healthy?* (Oxford, Oxford University Press, 2016), 31.

2 Seonaid Cleare et al., 'Self-compassion, Self-Forgiveness, Suicidal Ideation, and Self-Harm: A Systematic Review'. *Clinical Psychology and Psychotherapy* 26, no. 5, (2019): 511–30.

3 Andrew Bennett, *Suicide Century: Literature and Suicide from James Joyce to David Foster Wallace* (Cambridge: Cambridge University Press, 2017), 20.

4 Ian McWhinney, 'Being a General Practitioner: What It Means'. *European Journal of General Practice* 6 (2000): 135–39.

5 Ronald Epstein and Anthony Back, 'Responding to Suffering'. *Journal of the American Medical Association* 314, no. 24 (2015): 2623–24.

6 P Vergilius Maro, *Aeneid*, Book 1: 461–63.

7 Seamus Heaney, *Virgil's Poetic Influence*, an essay broadcast on BBC Radio 3 as part of the Greek and Latin Voices series, 15 July, 2008 (23:00).

8 Christopher Dowrick, 'Suffering and Hope: Helen Lester Memorial Lecture 2016'. *BJGP Open* 1, no. 1 (2017):bjgpopen17X100605.

9 Lori Montross Thomas et al., 'Yearning to Be Heard: What Veterans Teach Us About Suicide Risk and Effective Interventions'. *Crisis* 35, no. 3 (2014): 161–67.

10 Titus van Os et al., 'Communicative Skills of General Practitioners Augment the Effectiveness of Guideline-Based Depression Treatment'. *Journal of Affective Disorders* 84, no. 1 (2005): 43–51.

11 Stewart Mercer et al., 'Patient Enablement Requires Physician Empathy: A Cross-Sectional Study of General Practice Consultations in Areas of High and Low Socioeconomic Deprivation in Scotland'. *BMC Family Practice* 13, (2012): 6.

12 Stewart Mercer et al., 'General Practitioners' Empathy and Health Outcomes: A Prospective Observational Study of Consultations in Areas of High and Low Deprivation'. *Annals of Family Medicine* 14, no. 2 (2016): 117–24.

13 Jody Aked et al., *Five Ways to Wellbeing* (London: New Economics Foundation, 2011).

14 Christopher Dowrick et al., 'Get into Reading as an Intervention for Common Mental Health Problems: Exploring Catalysts for Change'. *Medical Humanities* 38, no. 1, (2012): 15–20.

15 Francis Bacon, *Study for a Portrait*, 1952: https://www.francis-bacon.com/artworks/paintings/study-portrait-0. Accessed 10 August 2021.

16 Edward Hopper, Automat, 1927: https://www.edwardhopper.net/automat.jsp. Accessed 10 August 2021.

17 Bertha Wegman, *Despair*, 1847–1926: https://pixels.com/featured/bertha-wegmann-danish-1847-1926-despair-bertha-wegmann.html. Accessed 10 August 2021.

18 Auguste Rodin, The Clenched Left Hand, c. 1885: https://www.metmuseum.org/art/collection/search/207496. Accessed 10 August 2021.

19 Alex Howick, 'Bristol Artist "Blown Away" By Reaction to Suicide Sculpture', BBC News Bristol, 6 April 2021: https://www.bbc.co.uk/news/av/uk-england-bristol-56654077. Accessed 9 August 2021.

20 Julia Bührle, 'Dances of Death from Paris to Saint Petersburg: Suicides in Ballet'. *European Drama and Performance Studies* 7 (2016):171–84.

21 Saxby Pridmore et al., 'Four Centuries of Suicide in Opera'. *Medical Journal of Australia* 199, no. 11 (2013): 783–86.

22 Ludwig Van Beethoven, *Violin Concerto*, performed by Itzhak Perlman with Daniel Barenboim and Berlin Philharmonic, 1992: https://www.youtube.com/watch?v=cokCgWPRZPg. Accessed 11 August 2021.

23 Quoted by Katie Mitchell, 'A Meeting of Minds', *The Guardian*, 18 November 2005: https://www.theguardian.com/music/2005/nov/18/classicalmusicandopera. thomasstearnseliot. Accessed 11 August 2021.

24 Robert Kahn, *Beethoven and the Grosse Fugue: Music, Meaning and Beethoven's Most Difficult Work* (Lanham: Scarecrow Press, 2010).

25 Tom Eames, 'The Story of ... "Staying Alive" by the BeeGees' *Smooth Radio* 18 September 2019. https://www.smoothradio.com/features/the-story-of/bee-gees-stayin-alive-lyrics-meaning-video/. Accessed 11 August 2021.

26 Michael Hainey, 'Beneath the surface of Bruce Springsteen' *Esquire*. 27 November 2018: https://www.esquire.com/entertainment/a25133821/bruce-springsteen-interview-netflix-broadway-2018/. Accessed 11 August 2021.

INDEX

A Long Way Down. *See* Hornby, Nick
Abrutyn, Seth 18, 23, 34, 43, 67
absurd 39, 65, 125
absurdity 49, 124, 125, 127, 132, 137
abuse 2, 21, 26, 27, 46, 50, 121
Achilles 76
adverse childhood events/experiences
    26, 118
agency 14, 106, 117, 121, 126
alcohol 6, 30, 50, 79, 90, 124, 126
alienation 14, 21, 67, 89, 106, 124,
    125, 133
altruism 11, 44
Alvarez, Al 15, 23, 47, 58, 74, 86, 88–90,
    93, 106–108, 113, 114, 124, 131
anamchara 106
ancient Egypt 86, 102, 104
Anna 13, 14, 18, 23, 24, 32–34, 37–52,
    55–59, 66, 86, 97, 102, 108, 112,
    114, 118, 131, 136, 138
Anna Karenina 37, 38, 51, 57–59, 102, 108,
    130, 131
    Leo Tolstoy 13, 14, 24, 32, 33, 37, 38,
    51, 55, 57–59, 86, 97, 102, 112, 114,
    130, 131, 136
anomie 14, 21
antidepressant medication 2
anti-natalism. *See* Benetar, David
anxiety 26, 34, 50, 119
anxiety and depression 50
Aristotle 9, 10, 18, 118, 129, 130
Armatrading, Joan 1
artistic creation 102
Ash Boughs 63, 72, 81
Attachment to the self 116
Ayres, Pam 93

Ba
    man and soul 104–107, 109, 112, 132
Bacon, Francis 136
Baldwin, James 138
Barnhofer, Thorsten 72
Barth, Karl 116
Bartlett, Rosamund 38
Bayne, Tim 117, 127, 129
Bearing witness 133
Beasley, Brett 71, 83
Beatles 137
Beckett, Samuel 57
BeeGees 137
bees 54, 123
Beethoven, Ludwig van 137
behavioural activation 53, 57
Benatar, David 113
Bennett, Andrew 13, 18, 91, 96, 97, 99,
    107, 108, 128, 139
bereaved by suicide 132
betweenpie 79
Billington, Josie 13, 17, 18, 38, 46, 48, 58,
    62, 81, 83, 107, 139
Black Sabbath's 137
bleak monotony 2, 71
bliss 98, 105
Bloom, Leopold 97, *See also* Joyce, James
Blum, Beth 10, 18
Born to Run. See Springsteen, Bruce
Bourne, Matthew 136
Bredin. Kathleen 122
Bridges, Robert 62, 65, 66, 68, 81–83,
    123, 129
Brodz, Ludek 122
Browning, Gary 46
Buber, Martin 116

Buddha 115, 129
Buddhist 68, 83, 94, 116, 127,
    See also Buddha
burden 26, 27, 46, 51, 68, 70, 88, 125
burdensomeness 27, 29, 33, 50
Burton, Robert 89

Camus, Albert 90, 124–127, 130, 132, 137
capability of suicide 50
Carrion Comfort' 65, 66, 73, 74, 83
Castano, Emanuele 11
catharsis 9, 40, 136, 138
Catholic 64, 94
chaos 66, 68, 96, 137
Charlie 1, 3, 10, 14, 20, 24, 29, 30, 38, 50,
    51, 56, 96, 121, 125, 131, 135–138
Chatterton, Thomas 89
Chekhov, Anton 12
Chobanov 106
choice to live 113
Christian 58, 59, 82
Christian anarchism 57
Chu, Carol 27
Cio-Cio-San. *See* Puccini
civic activism 133
civil liberties 138
climate change 30, 125
cognitive behavioural therapy 40
coherence 116, 118–120, 127
coherent beings 117
comfort 2, 3, 13, 32, 40, 51, 61, 64, 70, 71,
    73, 78, 79, 97, 113, 120, 121, 124,
    135, 138
common humanity 78
compassion 3, 4, 11, 13–15, 33, 49, 71, 78,
    79, 83, 88, 103, 107, 114–116, 124,
    127, 132–134, 136
compassionate 57, 78, 79, 83, 106, 136
compassionately. *See* compassion
connection 14, 33, 52, 64, 71, 74, 127, 135
Conrad, Joseph 119
consultations
    family doctor 6, 71, 134, 135
contemplation 13, 19, 20, 91
contingencies 49
continually completely new.
    See Strawson, Galen
cost of seriousness 86, 93

Costner, Kevin 44
courage 40, 74, 88, 91, 93, 132, 138
crisis 24, 30, 32, 47, 88, 90
cultural anthropology 19
curiosity 118
curtal sonnet 63, 72

Damastes (also known as Procrustes)
    Speaks. *See* Herbert, Zbigniew
Dancing in the Dark. *See* Springsteen,
    Bruce
Dante 89, 113
Darkness on the Edge of Town.
    See Springsteen, Bruce
Darren 2, 3, 10, 15, 27, 30, 120, 121,
    124–126, 128, 133, 134, 136–138
Davis, Philip 13, 18
Death 22, 34, 36, 73, 87, 91, 92, 101, 104,
    106, 114, 128, 129, 139
'death by soldiering' 44
death instinct 22, 23, 42, 88, 89, 91
deeply unconsolable 13, 33, 132
defeat 27–30, 33, 35, 42, 44, 47, 73, 136
defeated 14, 28, 47, 50, 51, 68, 73
defiance 73, 125
delight 62, 80
deliverance 49
denial of experience 90
deontology 114
depression 6, 20, 26, 28, 35, 53, 57, 59, 72,
    83, 89, 116, 134, 138, 139
depressive symptoms 11, 72, 79, 83
Descartes, Rene 118
desire 4, 6, 15, 23, 25, 26, 53, 74, 87, 89,
    101, 117, 118, 119, 121, 125, 127, 137
desire for survival 74, 119
desire to persevere 15, 117, 127
desolation 66, 69, 91
despair 2, 4, 10, 14, 19, 20, 24, 35, 39, 48,
    49, 51, 53, 55–57, 62, 66, 70, 73, 74,
    86, 89, 91, 102, 106, 107, 113, 115,
    119, 127, 131, 133, 136, 137, 139
desperation 48, 73
detachment 20, 72, 76, 96
determination 14, 73, 74, 90, 119,
    124, 131
Deus sive Natura. See Spinoza, Baruch
dignity 9, 31

dilemma 3, 14–16, 32, 38, 45, 51, 52, 55, 62, 73, 86, 102, 105, 107, 113, 126, 131, 133, 136–138
dilemmas of existence 8, 51, 57
distress 6, 8, 14, 28, 39, 41, 42, 47, 51, 53, 61, 68, 72, 81, 91, 96, 99, 106, 112, 127, 134, 135, 138
doctor-patient relationships 106
doctors. *See* family doctors
Dolben, Digby 62
Donne, John 89
Dubliners. See Joyce, James
dukkha 68, 115
Durkheim 14, 19, 20, 23, 24, 32–34, 42, 44, 58, 67, 82, 101, 108
Durkheim, Emile 19
Dying is 'the real aim of life'.
    See Schopenhauer, Arthur

Edmonds, Rosemary 38
egotistic
    suicide 42, 67
Eleanor Rigby. *See* Beatles
Eliot, George 97
    Middlemarch 12
Eliot, T.S. 137
empathy 11, 13, 71, 97, 99, 133, 134, 139
endeavour 119, 120
endurance 27, 33, 74, 86, 92, 114
endure 14, 27, 87, 92
engagement 13, 15, 53, 62, 104, 116, 122–124, 127, 132, 135
    and existential preservation 15
Engels, Frederick 64
entrapment 27–29, 33, 35, 47
    trapped 47
ephemeral 81, 98, 116
Epstein, Ron 116, 129, 139
escape, iii 4, 28, 47, 48, 50, 74, 107, 118
essence 33, 63, 74, 80, 104, 105, 114, 118–120
ethical existence 115
eudaemonia 122
evolutionary biologists 20
evolutionary biology 42
existential concerns 138
existential crisis 40, 66
existential dread 119

existential preservation 15, 54, 117
existential uncertainty 52, 56
existential unease 32, 36
existential weariness 74

faith 2, 7, 52, 71, 88
family doctor 6, 15, 27, 78
fear 1, 4, 9, 23, 26, 50, 91, 94, 119, 131–133
Felix Randal 64, 81, *See also* Hopkins
Fell
    multiple meanings 68
Five Ways to Wellbeing 135
flourish 1, 100, 107, 128
flourishing 15, 102
forgiveness 41, 42, 46, 49, 99, 133, 139
Forrest-Thompson, Veronica. *See* Porter, Peter
Frances 2, 3, 10, 14, 21, 30, 31, 57, 71–74, 76, 77, 79, 90, 133, 134, 136–138
freedom 21, 54, 125–127
Freud, Sigmund 14, 21–23, 33, 34, 42, 52, 58, 89, 91, 118
    mourning and melancholia 14, 22, 52, 89
futility of existence 97

Gandhi, Mahatma 56, 59
Garbo, Greta 38
Gask, Linda 8
general practitioners 134, 139
Ghosts 96
Giselle 136
Glendalough 79
glittering luminous core 81
God's fool 55
Goethe, Johann
    Werther 89
Gounod 136
grace 51, 99
gratitude 2, 62, 98
Greene, Graham 10, 107
Gregorius, Raimund 128
grief 2, 13, 15, 31, 37, 42, 51, 61, 68, 71, 85, 86, 89, 100, 102, 104, 106, 107, 115, 138
grieving 103, 126

Große Fuge. See Beethoven, Ludwig van
guilt 13, 44, 46, 89, 96, 99, 135

Haig, Matt, iii, 8, 10, 17, 18, 86, 94, 95,
    107–109, 132, 134
Hall, Joshua 74
Hamlet 15, 56, 73, 101, 112, 113, 127, 131
Hamnet. See O'Farrell, Maggie
happiness 8, 41, 46, 83, 90, 112, 116, 125
Hardwick-Smith, Robin 78
harm of existence 113
Harris, Daniel 66, 81, 82, 121–123
health professionals 57, 82, 133
Heaney
    Seamus 86, 91, 107, 132, 134, 139
Heath, Iona 94
Heiligenstadt Testament. *See* Beethoven,
    Ludwig van
hell 2, 67, 70, 89, 113, 121
Henley, William Ernest 76
Herbert, Zbigniew 86, 91, 107, 108
hieroglyphs 104
Homer 8
honesty 14, 71
hope 1, 6–8, 11, 15, 20, 32, 43, 48–51, 61,
    70, 73, 81, 90, 92, 94, 106, 107, 116,
    125, 132–134, 136–1389
hopelessness 31, 137
Hopkins, Gerard Manley 2, 4, 10, 13–16,
    20, 31, 33, 57, 61–71, 73–77, 79–83,
    86, 91, 92, 98, 108, 112–117, 120,
    121, 123–125, 127, 129–132, 135,
    137, 138
    Dublin 14, 33, 64, 67, 70, 82,
        87, 88, 123
    early life 62
    Liverpool 64
Hopper, Edward 136
Hornby, Nick 86, 94, 108, 123, 132
Hughes, Ted 88, 89
human existence 113–115, 128, 134
human meaning 13
humiliation 28, 33, 39–43, 47, 50,
    51, 57

I Wake and Feel 65, 66, 68–72, 77, 81
ideas of suicide 5, 15, 22
identity 23, 43, 67, 117, 120, 122, 137
Imagination 18, 119, 129

imagining suicide 133
inconstancy of language 100
ineffaceable 44
inexplicable 14, 101, 102, 107
Infinite Jest. See Wallace, David Foster
infinite possibilities of existence 132
injustices 121
inner mental subjectivity. *See* Strawson,
    Galen
inscape 63, 80, 81, 120, 128
instress 63, 80, 81
Integrated Motivational-Volitional Model,
    vii, 28
intentional action 117
intentional entity. *See* Bayne, Tim
interconnectedness 132
interdependence 122
Interpersonal Theory, vii, 25, 27, 34, 46
intersubjectivity 122, 128, 132
intractable conundrum' 99
Intuition 120
isolation 10, 23, 25, 30, 50, 51, 67,
    78, 97, 133
Ivbijaro, Gabriel 8

Joiner, Thomas
    Interpersonal Theory of Suicide 25–27,
        29, 34, 82
Jonah 75
Jones, Owen 138
joy 4, 54, 75, 78, 79, 81, 85, 98, 99, 118,
    138
Joyce, James 18, 32, 47, 86, 88, 89, 107,
    132, 139

Kagan, Annie 100
Karenin 41–46, 49
Keats, John 73, 83, 89, 135
Keen, Suzanne 11
Khomiakov 52
Kidd, David 11
Kierkegaard, Soren 112, 115,
    127–129, 132
kindness 70, 77, 78
King Lear 68, *See also* Shakespeare
Kirtley, Olivia 27–29, 35
Kitty 14, 38–40, 48, 51, 53, 55, 57, 102,
    123, 132, 135
Kitwood, Tom 122

languishment 4, 14, 65, 66
Larkin, Philip 89
legitimate 71, 135
Leigh 38, 86, 99, 100, 102, 132,
 132, 135
Lepsius, Karl 104
Levin 13, 14, 38, 43, 51–57, 66, 98, 112,
 114, 119–121, 123, 124, 131, 132,
 135, 138
liberation 116, 123, 125
Lichtheim, Miriam 104
literary activity 119
literary imagination 113
literary reading 2, 8, 10, 11, 13, 19, 53, 96,
 99, 107, 123, 131–137
literary reflections 113
literary texts 14, 15, 19, 32, 33,
 85, 107
literature
 destructive power 8
 healing power 8
loneliness 1, 4, 25, 27, 30, 35
Loyola, Ignatius 66

Macbeth 48, See also Shakespeare
Macfarlane, Robert
 Landmarks 13
MacIntyre, Alasdair 122, 130
Madama Butterfly. See Puccini
madeleine 118
Mantel, Hilary 6
Mariani, Paul 66, 81–83
Marx, Karl
 theories of alienation 14, 21, 32, 34
Marxian 67
Maude, Louise and Aylmer 38, 44, 57
McNeice, Louis 11
meaningless 41, 55, 97
meaninglessness 124
meditation 11, 72, 79, 116
memory 118
memory and emotion
 effects of literature 11
Menelaus 76
mental health 2, 3, 5, 6, 8, 11, 23, 30, 36,
 73, 123, 135
Merton, Robert
 strain theory 24, 47
Metaphysical solitude 52

Milbank, John 122
Miller, Hillis 66, 82
mindfulness 72, 78, 79, 83, 129
mindfulness meditation 72, 79
misery 39, 64, 103, 112, 114, 121
Mishima, Yukio 16
monotony 69,
Moorcock, Michael 1, 50, 96, 140
moral communities 122, 123, 127
moral purpose 54
Morrison, Toni 16
mortal sin 113
Mothering Sunday. See Swift, Graham
Mozart 10
Mueller, Anna 23, 34, 43, 58, 67, 82
multifarious possibilities 96
multiple selves 128
multiverses 95
Münster, Daniel 122
mutuality 122
My Own Heart 66, 81, 83, 130

Nabokov, Vladimir 46
narratives 16, 118
nausea
 Sartre 69
Neff, Kristin 78
negative thinking 72
negative thoughts 78, 79
new ways of being 106
Newman, John Henry 73
Nietzsche, Friedrich 8, 17
No Worst, There is None 61, 66, 68,
 81, 130
non-existence 19, 113, 121
non-violence 55
Norse sagas 102
North. See Heaney, Seamus
Not Waving but Drowning.
 See Stevie Smith

O'Connor, Rory 8, 17, 28, 29
 Integrated Motivational Model of
 Suicide. See Kirtley
O'Farrell, Maggie 20, 34, 86, 100–102,
 108
 Hamnet 20
Oates, Laurence 20
opium 47, 56

otherness 132
Owen, Wilfred 35, 89

Pabst, Adrian 122
Palach, Jan 32
pandemic 1, 5, 20, 30, 50, 51, 80, 121,
    125, 126
Papageno effect 10
paradox 86
Patience 66, 76, 77, 81–83
Pearson, Hilary 73, 82
perceived burdensomeness 25–27, 29
personal meaning 31, 52, 92, 121
personhood 32, 122, 130
Petrarch 62
Pevear, Richard 38, 44, 48, 52, 59,
    108, 130
Pichugin, Zahar 40
Piercey, Robert 12
Plath, Sylvia 49, 88–90, 93, 94, 113
Plato 8, 10, 18, 52
play 8, 9, 10, 29, 44, 63, 74, 88, 83, 94,
    101, 134, See also Porter, Peter
poetry and philosophy 9
Porter, Jannice. See Porter, Peter
Porter, Peter, viii, 74, 86, 93, 108, 113, 132
Portrait of the Artist as a Young Man.
    See Joyce, James
possibility of hope 50
potential 10, 15, 17, 57, 88, 92, 128
poverty 15, 28, 55, 121
power 7, 8, 10, 21, 32, 46, 55, 68, 114, 115,
    117, 119–121, 132, 134
practices. See MacIntyre, Alasdair
precarity 15, 88
Pridmore, Saxby 136
problem of suicide 6
Proust, Marcel 118
psychotherapy 2, 72
Puccini 136
punishment 48, 99

Rascal Flatts 99
reading groups
    impact on mental health 11
reasons to be 15, 113, 117, 123
reasons to stay alive 10, 33, 50, 95,
    106, 132
rebellion 126, 132

reciprocally-caring relationships 25,
    47, 50
reciprocity 122
refusal to surrender 73
regret 44, 47, 96, 135, 138
religion 13, 25, 99, 115
Religion 99
religious 4, 7, 13, 49, 52, 54, 55, 62, 81,
    86, 88, 89, 123, 127
religious belief 13, 127
remorse 44
resilience 29, 30
Resolution 98
resolve 15, 27, 33, 107
revenge 44, 104
revolt 43, 125, 127
Reyes-Foster, Beatrice 122
right action 123
Rodin, Auguste 136
Roland Smith, Robert 22
Romeo and Juliet 48
Rumi 2

sadness 4, 20, 42, 65, 68, 119
sanctuary 134, 138
Sands, Bobby 32
Sartre, Jean Paul 69, 82, 124, 126,
    130, 138
    Roads to Freedom 10
Savage God,. See Alvarez, Al
Schopenhauer, Arthur 52, 112, 114–116,
    120, 124, 127, 128, 131
Scotus, Duns 62, 63, 120, 132
self-destruction 21, 92, 95, 106, 123
self-destructive 47
self-harm 5, 6, 17, 26, 27, 29, 79, 133, 139
Self-kindness. See compassion
self-maintenance 119, 120
self-preservative 121
sense of coherence 15, 32, 117, 118,
    121, 127
sense of safety 68
    Lynch, Johanna 30, 33, 50, 52, 72
sense of self 1, 26, 30, 118, 121, 132
serious playfulness 92, 96
seriousness of living 15, 107, 132
Shakespeare 62, 91, 101, 102, 112, 113
    sonnet structure 62

shame 23, 31, 40–42, 44, 51, 57
Shange, Ntozake 16
shared experience 14, 71
Shelley, Percy Bysshe 89
Simpson, Joe 74
Sisyphus. *See* Camus, Albert
Skallagrimsson, Egil 102, 132
Smith, Stevie 15, 57, 74, 86, 91, 107, 108, 113, 114, 131, 132
Social
  connectedness 25, 132
  connections 20, 24, 26, 43
  contagion 29
  emotion 23
  integration 19, 67
  isolation 25
  justice 55
  network 18, 25
  psychology 19, 131, 132
  regulation 19
  relationships 30, 32
  world 23
solitude 69, 95, 98
Sonattorek. *See* Norse sagas
sonnet 62, 63, 65, 67, 70, 72–74, 76, 77, 80, 81, 123
sonnet therapy 62
sorrow 8, 61, 68, 69, 102, 115, 134
Spinoza, Baruch 52, 74, 83, 119–121, 125, 127, 128, 130–132
  conatus 74, 119, 120, 131
spiritual beliefs 52
spiritual good 132
spiritual understanding 54
Springsteen
  Bruce 137
sprung rhythm 63, 76
stay alive 3, 10, 14, 16, 19, 26, 38, 44, 51, 53, 55, 70, 72, 73, 103, 113, 114, 123, 126, 131, 132
Stayin' Alive. *See* BeeGees
staying alive 2, 5, 62, 113, 131
Stevenson, Juliet 91
strain 24, 25, 33, 82, 47, 52, 82, 67, 34
strain theory 47, 50
strains. *See* strain
Strakhov, Nicolai 43, 55, 58
Strawson, Galen 127, 128, 130, 132

Study to Deserve Death. *See* Stevie Smith
suffering 6, 20, 21, 26, 31, 39, 41, 43, 64, 67–70, 78, 79, 88, 102, 104, 106, 114–116, 127, 129, 133, 134, 137, 139
suicidal action 57
suicidal attempts 25
suicidal behavior 16, 19, 24, 27, 34, 35, 42
suicidal experience 33, 132, 133, 135, 137
suicidal ideas 5, 8, 14, 19, 25, 26, 28, 29, 32, 57, 66, 72
suicidal ideation 17, 25, 27–29, 32, 34, 35, 57, 79, 134
suicidal impulses 22, 42, 53
suicidal thinking. 72
suicidal thoughts 7, 23, 57, 131, 132, 135–137
suicidal thoughts and actions 23, 54, 131
suicide 4–8, 10, 11, 13–29, 32–35, 38, 40, 42–45, 47, 49–51, 53, 56, 58, 59, 70, 73, 74, 79, 82, 86–89, 91–93, 95–97, 99, 101, 104–106, 109, 112–114, 116, 121, 122, 124, 131–139
  baffling phenomenon 96
  definition 5
  impulsive act 49
  moral dimensions 56
  normalised activity 89
suicide as communicative act 32
suicide attempt
  overdose 1, 6, 50, 87, 95
suicide risk
  assessment by family doctor 6
  dimensions 6
  therapeutic strategies 7
suicide thoughts
  frequency 5
suicide, capability 26, 27
sunt lacrimae rerum 133, 134
Swan Lake 136
Swann's Way. See Proust, Marcel
Swift, Graham 86, 100, 108, 119
sympathy 49, 115
Szymborska, Wisława 93

Taylor, Charles 123, 130
Tchaikovsky, Piotr 61
tenacity 74

terrible sonnets 21, 62, 63, 66
The Aeneid. See Virgil
The Bottle of Aspirins. *See* Stevie Smith
The Cost of Seriousness. *See* Porter, Peter
The Midnight Library. See Haig, Matt
The Pale King. See Wallace, David Foster
The Red Shoes. See Bourne, Matthew
The Windhover 63, 80, 83, 108
theology of relationships 116
therapeutic connections 135
therapeutic encounters 15
therapeutic intervention 53
therapeutic literary resources 107
therapeutic potential 106
therapeutic strategies 132
Thomas, Chris 105
threats 4, 21, 30, 32, 47, 50, 52, 68, 73,
    92, 125
thwarted 46, 50, 51
thwarted belongingness 25–27, 33, 42, 46,
    50, 51, 68, 104
To Seem the Stranger 66, 72, 81
Tolstoy, Leo 3, 13–16, 22, 31, 37–39, 43,
    44, 48, 49, 51–59, 66, 86, 97, 98,
    108, 114, 115, 117–120, 123, 124,
    127, 128, 130–132, 137, 138
  Confession 58, 51, 16
  *The Kingdom of God Is Within
    You* 55
  What I Believe 55, 59
tragedy 8, 18, 112
transcendence 98
transformation 15, 85, 88, 92, 99, 102,
    106, 135
transformative 107
trapped 28, 30, 47, 51, 68, 74, 128
trauma 30, 40, 71
trust 16, 31
Two Lorries. *See* Heaney, Seamus

Ulysses. See Joyce, James
undefeated 76
univocity 62, 120, 128

Varenka 39, 40, 53, 57, 102, 132
Victoria Page. *See* The Red Shoes
Virgil 133, 134
visual and/or performing arts 15, 136
Vronsky 14, 24, 31, 32, 38–49, 59,
    57, 118
vulnerability/ies 1, 28, 29, 31

Wallace, David Foster 18, 86, 97, 98, 108,
    112, 131, 139
warrior 92, 126, 138
weary life 111, 112
webs of interlocution. *See* Taylor, Charles
Wegmann, Bertha 136
well-being 32, 36, 79, 112, 134
Weltschmerz 68
Werther fever
  Goethe 10
What *good* is done? *See* Bennett, Andrew
whirlwind 61, 70
White, Norman 66, 81, 82
Whitehouse, Amy 137
will to life 114, 127
Williams, Willam Carlos 12, 82, 86,
    101, 107
Woolf, Virginia 47
Wootten, William 3, 108
World Health Organisation 8, 16,
    17, 131
world in itself. *See* Schopenhauer, Arthur
wórld-sorrow 68

Zeldin, Theodore 119
Zhang, Jie 24, 25, 34, 47, 35, 59,
    67, 81
Zorin, Andrei 46, 55, 58

www.ingramcontent.com/pod-product-compliance
Lightning Source LLC
Chambersburg PA
CBHW020614270326
41927CB00005B/323